MAR 3 0 2009

Match Day

Match Day

One Day and One Dramatic Year
in the Lives of Three New Doctors

Brian Eule

St. Martin's Press
New York

www.stmartins.com

Library of Congress Cataloging-in-Publication Data

Eule, Brian.
    Match day : one day and one dramatic year in the lives of three new doctors / Brian Eule. — 1st ed.
        p. cm.
    ISBN-13: 978-0-312-37784-7
    ISBN-10: 0-312-37784-3
    1. Interns (Medicine)   2. Women physicians.   I. Title.
    [DNLM: 1. Internship and Residency—Personal Narratives.   2. Physicians, Women—Personal Narratives. W 20 E88m 2009]
    RA972.E95 2009
    610.92'2—dc22   2008042228

First Edition: March 2009

10   9   8   7   6   5   4   3   2   1

To S. D. C.

Contents

Match Day

Prologue

Some people held cups of coffee. Others held babies or the hands of spouses. David Kessler, the dean of the medical school, clutched a cell phone in one hand and a wireless e-mail device in the other. I clung to a small spiral notepad that listed family and friends we wanted to call when we got the news. And Stephanie, like every one of the other fourth-year medical students in the room, held an envelope.

The envelopes were brown and thin, each with a white label and a name on the front. A few minutes earlier, Dean Kessler had told the students to retrieve these envelopes by approaching one of the seven stations set up in the room. Although the students could pick up the envelopes, they were not to open them, he explained. "It's not time yet," he said, looking at his cell phone.

Stephanie had followed the dean's instructions and walked to a school employee sitting beneath a white sign that read A–CH. She quietly stated her name, "Stephanie Chao," and took the envelope handed to her. When she returned to me, she looked anxious for the first time that morning. "Let's get this show on the road," she whispered as she sat down. After holding the unopened envelope for a minute or two, she placed it on the table in front of us. Her long black hair, pulled tight in a ponytail, brushed against the back of her white sweater. She wore a bracelet of brown prayer beads on her wrist, "Buddha Beads," she called them, and it didn't hurt to have them with her on this day. Her mother had given her the bracelet when she was a teenager, and Stephanie put it on each morning when she got dressed. She didn't wear much other jewelry—if the prayer beads could even be called that. No rings on any of her fingers; just the bracelet, a petite watch, and a thin chain around her neck that I had given her after we started dating in college.

We sat inside the Golden Gate Room at her medical school, the University of California, San Francisco, on a March morning in 2006. A row of windows lined an entire wall of the room and through them, off in the distance, fog hid the choppy, uneasy waters of San Francisco Bay. To the left, the bridge for which the room was named towered above the low clouds and stretched more than eight thousand feet toward Marin, connecting the city to all possibilities north. To the right, the country unfolded east with Oakland, Denver, St. Louis, Chicago, Boston, New York— the real world, as my mother called it—lying just beyond the windows' frame.

Inside the room nearly 150 medical students and their loved ones waited. About half of the people sat at large round tables, while others crowded in the surrounding pockets of space. Almost all kept very still. One woman, standing in the corner, covered her face. Tears ran through her fingers and her body shook in anticipation. The man to her side placed his hand on her shoulder, but she didn't stop crying.

Most eyes in the room were fixed on Dean Kessler at the podium. The dean was a tall, thin man with a perfectly trimmed beard and hair neatly parted to the side. He checked the small screens on his cell phone and e-mail device for the exact time. During his tenure as the nation's commissioner of the Food and Drug Administration, Kessler had been a bit of a stickler, once overseeing the confiscation of more than two thousand cases of orange juice because the word *fresh* was included in the brand name, when in reality the juice came from concentrate. Now he wanted to make sure that UCSF's Match Day ran exactly according to the national protocol, and the fourth-year medical students gathering at school ceremonies across the country were not to open their envelopes until 9:00 A.M. Pacific Time, 10 A.M. Mountain, 11 A.M. Central, and noon Eastern. We still had five minutes.

Stephanie and I sat silently at the table. A year earlier, I had known nothing of this ritual. Foolishly, I had thought that if she and I decided to plan a life together, we would be able to pick where we wanted to live. She would apply for work and additional training as a doctor, just as I would look for a job after graduate school. We would weigh our options and make a decision. But for the past year, as I learned more about the Match and as it occupied more of my thoughts, I knew it wouldn't happen quite like that. Stephanie's future, which in all likelihood meant my own, as well as the futures of more than fifteen thousand fourth-year medical students across the country, would all be dictated at the exact same moment.

Although these students were still a few months from the

crowning ceremonies in which they would officially be pronounced doctors, this day—Match Day—seemed a more important culmination. They had each selected a field of medicine, then spent months working on applications and interviewing at hospitals. After the interviews, they ranked an order of preference for the hospitals in which they hoped to have their first jobs as doctors during the post–medical school period known as residency. The hospitals made similar ordered lists of their favorite candidates. Then, in the final step of the process, a computer in a Washington, D.C., office ran an algorithm that paired each student with a residency position. Each year on Match Day, at the same time across the country, the graduating students are handed their envelopes. Inside, a fragment of a sentence on a single sheet of paper dictates their first job as a doctor—and thus, their careers. The right job in the right program might open the door to prestige, power, and happiness. The right city might make it easier for a spouse or partner to tag along. But the wrong words on that sheet of paper could lead a person down a path of heartache.

This is the ritual every year. But there was something unique about the medical students in the room with us on this day, and those across the country waiting for the same minutes to pass; something different from the gatherings that had made up Match Days in earlier years, and part of an evolving trend. While about 72 percent of all practicing physicians in the United States were men, the room seemed evenly made up of male and female medical students. Across the country the same statistic held true—nearly 50 percent of the nation's medical graduates were women. Entering a field in which they would be required to work years of eighty-hour weeks and multiple overnight shifts, these women were forced to consider how to balance their careers and any desire to have children—a desire they often felt the need to hide on residency interviews—all before their careers even began, all in advance of this one day. Such considerations were not completely new; the handful of women who had entered the profession in years prior had also faced these challenges. But medicine was deeply rooted in tradition, and with this new generation, the face of medicine was changing along with many of its ways.

Three minutes remained. As we waited for the dean's green light, I felt my heart step up the pace through my thick black sweater. I was neither a doctor nor a medical student, but I knew my future was at stake, especially as I debated proposing to Stephanie in the next year. When I had met her in college, five years earlier, she kept a shelf full of books on the MCAT, the entrance exam for medical school, and had no doubts about wanting to become a doctor. She also had about the biggest smile I had ever seen. Around the same time, I considered a career in journalism, though I had recently shied away from my boyhood idea of covering a baseball team after talking to a sportswriter about the 162-game season, half of which took place on the road. He was unshaven and a bit on the heavy side. I asked him how was it to be gone from his family for such long periods of the year.

"I don't have a family," he told me.

Oh, I said. Was it something he ever considered, or was it too difficult with the job?

"Listen," he told me. "I have to have a job. I don't have to have a family. I might as well love my job."

I wanted both. Stephanie said that she did too. She went straight from college to medical school with the understanding that she had a long road ahead of her and that if she wanted to have children, she had better get her training out of the way as quickly as possible. She loved how her own mother had been so present in her and her siblings' lives when they were young, taking them on excursions to the park and making their lunches for school. Family was crucial to Stephanie. But in the last few years she had also grown attached to the field of surgery. Balancing children with career was difficult for the few women in this demanding and predominantly male-populated specialty. Surgery would require a seven-year intensive residency at the hospitals she had applied to, followed by another few years of a fellowship if she chose to specialize, and finally, a lifetime of an all-consuming job.

Two more minutes.

I knew that some of the possibilities in Stephanie's envelope could mean a more difficult life than others. A hospital she had interviewed with in Boston was known for great training, but also for eliminating any kind of an outside life for the seven years of residency. Although the hours at one of the programs in California would not be much better, we had heard that at least some of its residents had families. Rumors swirled on the interview trails. One small program, we were candidly told, had a divorce rate among its residents of more than 100 percent. I asked how that was possible. Someone got married and divorced twice, a resident told me.

The nervous chatter in the room continued. We sat above the university's fitness center on the section of campus dedicated to recreation. A cafeteria bordered us on one side with a table-tennis room for students on the other. Across the street, separated from Match Day by two lanes of traffic, a circular driveway, and parked ambulances, lay the university's hospital. Nationally recognized doctors, overtired residents, nurses, therapists, and students swirled down halls and in and out of patients' rooms. Lives began. Lives ended. In just over three months the halls would be filled with new interns—the colloquial term for first-year residents, the rookie doctors. My father, who had been a frequent hospital patient, had always warned me about this time. "You don't want to get sick in July," he said. A teaching hospital is a wonderful place to get care, and it's where you find the best doctors in the country, but in late June and July, you also find a lot of people who don't know what they're doing.

One minute remained.

In the months leading up to Stephanie's Match, I found myself fascinated by this process for pairing new doctors with their new lives, and by the challenges the next generation of doctors faced as the profession reshaped. But most of all, I wondered about how Stephanie's life, and thus mine, was about to change. The next year would be a trial of sleepless nights, beeping pagers, and demanding senior physicians.

We looked at the dean. We looked at the envelope. Stephanie turned to me. "Do you want to be the one to open it?" she asked.

Someone called time.

1

The Matchmaker

For a few minutes, in the weeks before medical schools began the nerve-racking ceremonies of handing out envelopes, 15,008 graduating students from U.S. allopathic medical schools were jammed into a single room in the northwest quadrant of Washington, D.C. They did not appear in person, clutching résumés or transcripts. Their essays and letters of recommendation were nowhere in sight. They, and their list of preferences, arrived only as computerized data points. Everything that mattered had been reduced to a few numbers for this final step. That way, a simple desktop computer running MatchPro software could pair each applicant with the teaching hospital where he or she would spend the next three-to-seven years of training. Nothing about the computer, or the desk on which it sat, seemed special. The only indication of all the lives altering course at that very moment was the series of numbers briefly displayed on the computer's monitor.

The Match had numbers for everything. Medical students

entered their eight-digit identification codes on the Match's Web-based "Registration, Rankings, and Results System." Historic institutions were coded with four digits. Harvard's Massachusetts General Hospital became 1261. Johns Hopkins, 1241. The Mayo Clinic in Minnesota, 1328. A series of three numbers indicated the specialty a new doctor would practice. A career in anesthesiology meant the numbers 040. General surgery was coded as 440. Dermatology, 080. Combined, strings of numbers formed the genomes of the thousands of residency programs with positions for the nation's newest doctors.

The computer worked efficiently. It made temporary matches based on the first student and hospital rank order lists it came across, then reassigned the candidates as it digested more lists, shifting future doctors like contestants in a high-speed game of musical chairs. By the time the music stopped, the computer program had married the majority of the country's newest doctors to the hospitals where they would first practice medicine. The actual matching took less than ten minutes. It was over before most people knew it began.

A few other computers ran similar operations for a small handful of medical specialties. It was the urology match that caused panic one year with an onslaught of undesirable results until the American Urological Association revealed that there had been a glitch in the computer system and its match would be run again. For the vast majority of students, though, it was the computer in the National Resident Matching Program's office that held their results in its digital pairings. The staff carefully checked the data several times, uploaded the results into a password-protected online system, and prepared reports. But it would be days before the students would learn the results.

First came the Monday before Match Day—the day students dubbed "Black Monday." Applicants raced to Internet connections and logged into the online system to learn whether or not they matched. No other details were given. On average, the computer only spit out 6 or 7 percent of the country's allopathic medical school seniors—the students who would be awarded the M.D. degree—without a position. Often they had applied in a competitive field and not ranked enough hospitals. The numbers weren't always as favorable for the thousands of independent applicants—a group that included graduates of foreign medical schools and osteopathic schools. The wrong news on Black Monday meant moving on to the Scramble—a frantic two-day process in which unmatched students, with the help of their deans, telephoned programs with unfilled positions and tried to sell themselves. But for the majority, seeing the words "Congratulations, you have matched!" meant a quick sigh of relief, then waiting three more days for a ritual that had grown more intense and anticipated than graduation itself.

On the third Thursday in March, medical schools across the country held gatherings to unveil the computer's results. Some schools waited for the designated hour, then unleashed the students to retrieve the envelopes with their results and braced for a stampede. Others, including Vanderbilt University, called students at random to the front of a lecture hall. On the way, each student dropped a dollar bill into a fishbowl as compensation for the suffering that the last person was to endure while waiting. One by one, they received and opened their envelopes, leaned into a microphone, and announced the result to classmates, family, and anybody watching on Vanderbilt's live Webcast.

Students could skip the ceremonies and wait to view results

online later in the day, but it was a harrowing process no matter how the medical school or student treated the day. Some students misunderstood the way the computer worked and wondered if they could game the system by altering their rank lists. Others finished interviews with winks from program directors or post-interview phone calls, like high school basketball stars recruited by overzealous college coaches, and were stunned if they did not match with a particular hospital. The not-for-profit National Resident Matching Program, which, as it described itself on its Web site, provided "an impartial venue for matching applicants' and programs' preferences for each other consistently," could show the Match as a success for the masses, with more than 80 percent of the candidates ending up at one of their top three choices. Yet for the individual applicant, suddenly embarking on a new career at a different, less appealing institution than hoped for could be hard to cope with; leaving students sometimes wondering about the origins of this unusual process.

After twenty years of exams and classrooms, the fourth-year medical students were just a few months shy of commencement ceremonies in which they would suddenly be pronounced doctors. Years of bending over Robbins's Pathology and Netter's Anatomy textbooks, inhaling formaldehyde seeping from dissected cadavers, and writing ever-growing tuition checks gave way to jobs and legitimacy. But while deans and diplomas could transform students into physicians, a new doctor lacked sufficient experience. As a result, since the early 1920s, a postgraduate year of intense on-the-job training had been standard practice. For physicians who wanted to specialize, that training formalized into from three to seven years, depending on a doctor's desired specialty. This extended training period was called residency. The first year was internship.

When internship and residency were first developed, the young doctor lived at the hospital, hence the term *resident,* and expectations of a life devoted solely to work were hinted at, with some hospitals forbidding marriage. Interns were allowed to practice medicine under a hospital's license. They weren't paid much, if anything, were sleep deprived, and had few days off. Though most interns no longer live at the hospital, the practice continues today. The weak are toughened, hospitals get the help they need at a cheap price, and new doctors are initiated into the world of medicine with the experience and patient care time they require.

But soon after the development of the internship, fierce competition for the best graduating medical students led to problems. With more positions than candidates, some hospitals raced to offer internships before their competitors. At first, they contacted fourth-year medical students, but soon reached out to third-years, more than a year in advance of the job. By the 1940s, some students reported receiving offers in their second year of medical school, despite the fact that hospitals could only guess, at such an early point, who would turn out to be the best doctors.

To stop this trend and the disruption it caused, the Association of American Medical Colleges agreed that schools would not release transcripts and recommendations until after a student's third year of medical school. While this tactic worked in pushing back the date of the offers, it led to another problem. Now hospitals limited the time a student had to respond to an offer, hoping to avoid being left with a shortage of doctors should a candidate take too long to reply with a rejection. Students were given ten days to respond. They complained of pressure and often accepted the first position to come along, only to regret the decision or consider rescinding it if a better offer arrived. By then, a hospital might have lost out on its second, third, or fourth choice. The following year, students were given only seven days to respond. The year after, it was three. One year later, students had twelve hours.

Again, the association worked on a solution, this time convening a committee to work on a centralized clearinghouse as the final step in the selection process. Students would still apply to and interview at hospitals. But by submitting an ordered list ranking their choices at the conclusion of the interview season, they were not pressured or rushed into accepting an offer. And hospitals, with their own ordered lists of applicants who had interviewed, had no need to fear the repercussions of a student's rejection. After a trial run during the 1950–51 school year, and altering of the algorithm when a group of students pointed out that it could penalize those who listed unrealistic first choices, the process was agreed upon and implemented the following year. The Match, as it was called, proved a popular solution and more than fifty years later was still in effect. Though like a living organism, it had changed over the years.

If you wanted to put a face on this faceless machine, it would have a thick black beard, beginning to go gray. It would have a receding hairline. It would wear glasses, squint when smiling, and present a big forehead adding to its contemplative appearance. It would look, in this case, much like an economist at Harvard University named Alvin Roth.

For his fiftieth birthday, colleagues crowned Roth with a hat that read, "Mr. Matching." He fit the stereotypical image of a professor, pacing the classroom when he spoke to a group, his conversations and lectures rich with hypotheticals and examples of conundrums. By the time I grew interested in the Match, Roth's algorithms assigned children to schools in Boston, placed teenagers at New York City public high schools, selected compatible kidneys and patients for transplants in a process known as paired donations, and since 1998, ran on the National Resident Matching Program's computer. Despite this, Roth remained unrecognizable to most physicians. He rarely even mentioned his work on personal checkups or encounters with doctors. It was the medical students' scores, interview skills, and rank order lists that led to their jobs, he told people, not his algorithm. The way he viewed it, he had simply been a consultant hired to fix a marketplace that had grown controversial again.

As a young assistant professor of economics at the University of Illinois in the early 1980s, Roth had called up the school's medical librarian and asked for any articles on the Match. He was full of curiosity. The unique process had handled the labor market for doctors for thirty years, and Roth wanted to see what made it work. By an economist's terms, he decided, the Match's success had to do with stability: there was no hospital and candidate not already matched to each other in which both parties wished they were. That seemed important—if the Match had been unstable, Roth figured, it would have led hospitals and candidates to circumvent the system.

The algorithm functioned somewhat like a common mathematical equation taught in schools known as the stable marriage algorithm. When Roth first studied the Match, its algorithm started with the hospitals' rank lists or, as some described it, with the hospitals proposing to the students. The students matched with their top choices among the offers they received. Roth wrote several papers on the process and in 1990 coauthored an academic book called *Two-Sided Matching: A Study in Game-Theoretic Modeling and Analysis.* By 1995, the National Resident Matching Program called him for help.

It seemed the Match had come under some scrutiny. In an article for *Academic Medicine,* a Philadelphia medical professor accused the National Resident Matching Program of not clearly portraying the algorithm as favoring the hospitals. He also wondered whether, under the current system, students had incentives to misrepresent their preferences on their rank list to improve their chances. Students wondered whether they were at a disadvantage because they were not the ones proposing in the algorithm. The Health Research Group—a division of a consumer advocacy group formed by Ralph Nader—and the American Medical Student Association prepared a report on the alleged hospital bias in the Match, and sent a letter of concern to the Association of American Medical Colleges requesting that the algorithm be switched from hospital-optimal to student-optimal.

If people were concerned about the Match, they might stop using it. And if some stopped, the system would break down for the rest. So the National Resident Matching Program hired Roth to study the existing algorithm and create one in which the students proposed. Complicating the situation were all the variations the Match now took into account. Some students needed to submit two separate lists—one for an intern year and one for the remaining years of residency—if their residency program didn't include the internship as part of its training. Other students applied to the Match as a couple, linking their lists together.

The National Resident Matching Program gave Roth and a fellow consultant, Elliott Peranson, five years of Match data. Roth experimented with alterations to the algorithm like a kid playing with a chemistry set, testing to see how different actions caused new reactions. He changed the algorithm and sent it off to Peranson to plug in, then watched as some of the candidates—their names and identifying information blocked out—paired with different hospitals than they had in the real Match.

Roth got a kick out of what he was doing, but he denied that he was playing with lives. He was just exploring possibilities, moving numbers around, and altering the order of the operation. On occasion, he got visits from an officer of the American Medical Student Association, or a hospital's program director, and Roth suspected they were feeling him out to see if he was in the pocket of the other guys. "Look, I'm an economist," he told them. To prove it, he launched into long orations about the intricacies of the algorithms. Visitors might walk away baffled but oddly satisfied.

Ultimately, Roth found that for either algorithm—the existing one or his new one—applicants and residency programs would have the best results if they played by the rules and arranged their lists simply by preference rather than shorten lists or change their first choices. He also discovered that the new algorithm, in which students proposed, helped a very small number of additional applicants—about one in a thousand— earn spots at institutions higher on their lists. Still, the National Resident Matching Program adopted Roth's new algorithm, and it was in the computer by 1998. The controversy over, things seemed calm for a few years.

But there was another concern that had never been addressed. The Match, some students complained, left candidates with no power to negotiate. Although students applied to hospitals and went on interviews, much like candidates in any job market, the Match meant the graduating students most in demand did not have multiple offers to use to negotiate salary and employment conditions. The free market was eliminated. Students signed binding agreements on entering the Match, and thus candidates had little choice but to accept the conditions of the hospitals with which they matched. On average, the $43,000 annual salary for a doctor just out of medical school was less than half that of a recent law school graduate at some large private firms and translated into a wage of approximately ten dollars an hour. After taking on hundreds of thousands of dollars in medical school loans, these young doctors needed all the money they could get.

In 2002 a resident and two former residents filed an antitrust lawsuit against dozens of teaching hospitals and seven professional associations, including the National Resident Matching Program, claiming that the Match kept wages low and hours long by denying them the right to negotiate. Some viewed the suit as having no merit and noted that the Match didn't affect wages. Roth pointed out that the wages for fellows—a step after residency for doctors who wished to further specialize—were unrelated to a match. A number of fellowships used a match and others did not, yet the salaries were comparable.

Still, the legal process dragged on, and each year the mystery around the Match grew. New medical students learned of the

Match only to wonder if it would still be in effect by their fourth year of medical school. By 2004, Congress passed legislation tacked on at the bottom of a pension funding equity act to ensure the Match's protection. "Antitrust lawsuits challenging the matching process, regardless of their merit or lack thereof, have the potential to undermine this highly efficient, pro-competitive, and long-standing process," it stated, concluding that the act would ensure that antitrust laws would not prohibit a graduate medical education residency matching program. Citing the new law, a federal court ultimately threw out the case.

For the students who entered medical school just months after the lawsuit began, that meant the match would spit out results for them on the most climactic day of medical school, just as it had for fifty-four graduating classes before them. They were the medical school class of 2006 and, among the thousands of eight-digit identification codes, there was one that made the whole process very personal for me.

Forty miles north of the desktop computer, Baltimore was a city attempting to reinvent itself. Yellow tower cranes stood watch over construction by the harbor, and billboards and banners greeted us at almost every corner with one word—Believe. It seemed to be a marketing campaign for the city, though without any other words on the signs, I was not sure what it was the city wanted me to believe. We walked in the crisp evening, not far from the hotel where Johns Hopkins University's Department of Surgery was hosting a reception for its interview candidates that evening, and I held Stephanie's hand. Four months remained until Match Day.

The evening's reception was open to spouses and partners,

and Stephanie had suggested I come along, though now she wondered how to introduce me. Boyfriend, she said, didn't seem to do our relationship justice. We had dated longer than some of our friends who were already married. But long-term boyfriend sounded a bit wordy. And with no ring on her finger, she didn't want to lie and call me her fiancé.

I looked at Stephanie and a slow grin formed on my face. "I don't want to have to remedy the situation right now," I said. She smacked me across the arm.

"I could just not introduce you at all," she said. "Or maybe I should just say, 'This is my friend.'"

I laughed. That's how her mother once presented me to several extended members of their family when we first started dating. She had said something in Chinese and everybody smiled and nodded. Stephanie had giggled and whispered in my ear. "She just told them, 'This is Stephanie's friend, Brian.'"

I told Stephanie not to worry about introducing me to the surgeons. If anyone asked, I would respond that I wasn't a medical student and that I was here with Stephanie. I knew that tomorrow she would try to impress the department's doctors during five separate interviews. But tonight, before all that began, it was the department's turn to paint the residency program as attractively as possible. This did not seem a difficult task. Johns Hopkins was constantly ranked the best medical center in the country, and its tradition of training top-notch surgeons was rich. Still, other students had told Stephanie there was more to the intricate dance of interview, rank, match. If a visit convinced her to rank a program high, word was, she should write its directors a letter letting them know, or maybe even have a department chair from her medical school make a phone call on her behalf. Ideally, the Match was supposed to make the whole process straightforward. It added order and was intended to lead to student and program rank lists that were made independently of each other. But whispers among students spoke of residency directors who liked to know who was most interested in their program so they could rank the candidates accordingly and brag about not having to go low on their own rank list.

Inside the Baltimore hotel, circular tables filled the conference room. A small table in the back held some drinks. Another held a tray of crab dip. Two or three dozen people milled about the room. We sat at a table with two tired-looking residents and a couple of wide-eyed candidates. Somebody asked one of the residents what he thought of Baltimore.

"It's a shitty city," he said. An awkward laugh rose from the candidates.

"Really, I'm not joking," he said. But the fact that the hospital was in such a bad neighborhood was a good thing, he went on to say, claiming that Johns Hopkins residents saw more penetrating trauma—all of those stab wounds and gunshot victims—than almost any other hospital. After a residency at Johns Hopkins, a surgeon would feel competent operating on any case. Stephanie leaned forward. When he added that he had been mugged while walking home one night, she gave me a quick glance. Then she turned her attention back to the resident.

I excused myself to get a drink. Another group of people chatted by the bar, and one woman introduced herself as the wife of a resident. She admitted that a surgical resident's lifestyle wasn't great. Hours were long. Emergencies occurred in the middle of the night. Schedules were unpredictable. I asked if it was hard on her. She smiled. "I knew what I was getting into," she said.

Stephanie liked to tease me that I didn't know what I was in for when we started dating. We were college students. She had told me she wanted to go to medical school and that she thought she might become an oncologist or a pediatrician. It wasn't until after we met that she decided to become a surgeon—the medical specialty that, I came to realize, had one of the longest and most grueling residencies.

We met on the third floor of a dormitory on the south side of Stanford's campus. I had drawn a terrible number in the university's housing lottery for my senior year, landing a room in Trancos, a dormitory filled with freshmen and a few other unlucky lottery losers. Stephanie's room was two doors down. She was a junior, there to serve as the head academic adviser for the students, or H.A.A., as they were called. Everything at Stanford was shortened to an acronym or lazy nickname. Memorial Church became MemChu. A visiting prospective freshman was a ProFro. And Stephanie was the H.A.A.

I often ran in and out of the dormitory, off to visit friends or check in at the student newspaper where I worked, and during the first few days of the year, I got sidetracked on my way out. Stephanie left her door open in case the freshmen needed any help. I'd stop in her doorway, tell her a joke or two, and try to get her to laugh. "Did you hear the one about the three guys who went up to heaven?" I asked. When she shook her head no, my heart started beating fast and I did my best not to ruin the joke. At one point, my roommate saw me eyeing Stephanie as she walked down the hall.

"Well, well," he said.

"Oh, it's nothing," I told him.

He gave me a smile. "Right," he said.

She was tall, with long, dark hair and a smile so frequent that I could close my eyes and still see the pink above her teeth peeking out from her lips. It made me want to do anything just to get a laugh from her. After college, we both lived in San Francisco, and I drove her around in my Buick, a white, boxy car. A retired chemistry professor had donated it to a community center that turned around and sold the automobile to me for just over a grand. It had a dead battery, broken alternator, and small black knob that kept slipping off the end of the gearshift. The night after I replaced the battery and alternator, I took Stephanie for a ride, cruising around our neighborhood and serenading her with radio songs sung into the black knob, which I put to my lips, throwing in a Sinatra-style "Hey!" or "Yeah!" between beats. I turned to her, at a red light, smiling, waiting for a response to my new wheels, prompting her with an "Eh?" and raised eyebrows. She laughed, then told me the car rode smoothly, like a taxi, and leaned in under my arm.

Stephanie was the child of Chinese immigrants, and she spoke with pride whenever she mentioned how her father once sold toothbrushes door-to-door to make ends meet. But she laughed when anyone asked her if her parents had pressured her to go to medical school. If anything, they tried to talk her out of it.

When Stephanie was born, her parents, shrewd business-people, owned a restaurant on Pier 39. It had been purchased shortly before the area became San Francisco's hottest tourist point. Her mother and father worked together—first at the restaurant, then at other ventures—and dinner conversations often involved work. Young Stephanie soaked it in. As a child, she crafted business cards out of construction paper, scribbled her name, and toted them around the house in her father's briefcase.

But when Stephanie announced in high school that she was considering a career in medicine, her mother looked concerned. A doctor's life was a difficult one, her mother told her. It was an important profession and wonderful if Stephanie decided to devote her life to work, her mother said, but it would be very hard to be a good doctor and a good mother. How would Stephanie feel if she was called into the hospital in the middle of the night while her own child was home sick with a fever? Her mother wasn't saying that a woman couldn't have a career and a family—she herself had juggled caring for three children with full-time work. It just seemed less plausible as a doctor. Stephanie said her mother was wrong. She could do it. Lots of people did it, she said. (And as lead prosecutor on the high school's mock trial team, Stephanie knew how to argue.)

So her mother suggested Stephanie try shadowing a doctor for a little while. She expected the experience would discourage the teenager. But she misjudged her daughter—Stephanie loved it. One day each week, just weeks after she earned her driver's license, Stephanie drove to a cardiologist's office in San Francisco. She followed the doctor from the sink, where he scrubbed his hands, to the patients' rooms, where he listened to complaints with compassion. She watched as nurses and other doctors came to him with questions and he made confident decisions on the spot. She was enamored with the profession. By the time we met in college, she had aced the Medical College Admissions Test, two years before she would go to medical school.

As a medical student, she loved any time in the operating room—"Here, Stephanie, hold the liver out of the way," a surgeon once told her. She put her gloved hand in the patient and spread her fingers around the organ. It felt thick, like a raw chicken breast but warm, and she pushed it back and watched the surgeon cut. Before surgery, a patient had a problem. After, the problem was fixed. The change was tangible and Stephanie liked that.

I knew I got to see a different, sillier side of Stephanie than her classmates or professors. In the quiet of her apartment, she was playful. Some days, she entered a room dancing for no apparent reason, kicking her arms and legs out to the side. Other evenings, she might suddenly race toward me with arms stretched forward, yelling, "Piiiiink belly!" At the onset of her war cry, I had to figure out an escape route or my stomach would get a pounding. There was no question she brought vivacity to everything she did in life. But her medical school professors and classmates saw a more professional side—an elegant and polite woman. She was the kind of student who could leave you either annoyed or dumbfounded by making success look effortless. She organized a series of lectures called Real Medicine, where students heard from guests about the variety of ways a medical degree could be put to use. She volunteered to teach an elective on medical Mandarin language. And she impressed the doctors on her clinical rotations at the hospital. When the university wrote letters evaluating the graduating students, it classified them by way of an adjective—outstanding, followed by superior, excellent, very good, or good—depending upon how many honors the students received on their medical school rotations. Stephanie's nine honors were enough to lead the university to tout her as outstanding. She seemed a strong candidate for any residency program.

Still, if a candidate didn't interview at enough places, the chances of matching decreased. Most of the students who received bad news on Black Monday ranked, on average, only five hospitals. The number of programs on a rank list for a matched student was closer to eight. Stephanie decided to apply to fifteen surgical residency programs around the country. Even if they all invited her to interview, she would probably only visit and rank eight. Between plane tickets and hotels, the residency interview season could cost a medical student thousands of dollars. In addition to Baltimore, she lined up dates in Philadelphia, Boston, North Carolina, and Northern and Southern California, and had already completed an interview in Missouri. Both of our families lived in California, and once, before either one of us knew about the Match, we had talked about how we could imagine calling the San Francisco Bay Area home. But now that plan seemed up in the air.

In fact, just about everything in my life seemed that way. I was more serious than just a boyfriend. Not yet a fiancé. After a short stint as a newspaper reporter following college, I was no longer sure what I wanted to do with my career. While Stephanie finished her last two years of medical school, I had left to attend graduate school in a writing program on the other side of the country. I contorted my six-foot-three body onto a twin mattress in a rented New York bedroom during the school year and found work in San Francisco in the summer to be with her. I was twenty-seven years old. Though I was only months away from finishing the graduate program, I was unsure what I would do for a job. And it was difficult to plan for a future because, if I wanted that future to be with Stephanie, I had no idea where it would be.

One day my mother pulled me aside. She told me that if I ever wanted to, I could use her engagement ring. It wasn't a perfect stone, she said. It had a crack on the edge somewhere. But it was what my father had given her, and she thought I might like that.

I grew up knowing that my father was madly in love with my mother. They met when he was seventeen years old and she was eighteen, both in their first year of college at the State University of New York at Stony Brook. The way my father told the story, he knew he wanted to marry my mother from the moment he saw her. He was at a party in the lounge of their college dormitory. He sat on a couch and propped his broken leg up on a coffee table. In front of him, two cheerleaders stood talking. In the space between them, he saw my mother, standing across the room. Right then and there, he knew she was the one he wanted to marry. My mother turned to me when she heard this story. "That's ridiculous," she said. "There's no way he knew."

They were engaged shortly after graduation, and my father went upstate to begin law school. My mother followed him to Ithaca, then back to New York, to Rochester, to Boston, to Philadelphia, and to California. My father's career dictated where the family lived. My mother stayed at home with my sister and me when we were young, then took a job as a dental office manager.

My father was a wonderful storyteller, even if he did embellish at times. But of all the stories, cancer was the biggest. It was like a war story for him—an enemy he was proud to have defeated when I was just three years old. A doctor gave him an 11 percent chance of surviving his lymphoma, and somehow he did. I didn't remember him being sick, but I saw the effect it had on his life. Family came first. Each day was one more than he expected. He left work early for basketball games and school plays. He was a Jewish man whose voice gave away his New York roots, but when he drove our morning car pools, he bellowed, "Top of the morning," to me and my friends in his best attempt at an Irish accent. And he wouldn't start driving until we replied, "And the rest of the day to you," as he had instructed us on so many occasions.

But when I was seventeen, around the time of my parents' twenty-fifth anniversary, I learned that my father was going back to war. This time, the images of his struggle with cancer burned into my memory. The hospital's sterile halls became familiar, though never warm. Strangers in white coats entered and exited the room, and with them, grief and hope. I looked up each time, searching for clues in their faces before they could open their mouths. I watched a neurosurgeon's walk, step by step, as he met us in the lobby one morning, though I turned away before his departure. Six months after my father died, I left for college.

My mother didn't know what to do with the ring. For a while, she continued to wear it. Then she had the stone placed in a different setting, to look less like an engagement ring. But if I ever wanted it, she told me, it was mine. I thanked her and asked her to hold on to it until I needed it one day.

For many, the two great matches of a person's life were playing out at the same time. If the only concern on Match Day was to get the best professional training, there didn't seem much to mope about if the computer printout listed a choice other than your number one. Young doctors could receive solid training at many institutions. While living in New York might be hard for a Red Sox fan, there wasn't much time to go to a ball game anyway. But everything became more complicated when you factored in another reality: many of these people were making decisions about family. Dating, relationships, engagements, even fragile young marriages were at stake. Heading to an unexpected city could determine which romantic relationships blossomed into lifelong partnerships and which burned out or simply withered away.

With more women in medicine, and thus more medical school romances, the Match had made a technical nod at the problem of two medical students going through the process together. It offered an option on the rank list in which two doctors could designate a couple's match. But this only brought about additional stress as medical students were forced to decide, were they a couple or not?

In that year before the 2006 Match, I spent much of my time on the other side of the country from Stephanie, thinking about our future. It eased the loneliness to know that my close friend Aaron was also in New York, finishing medical school. Through Aaron, I found a circle of friends in his classmates from New York Medical College. My own classmates had never heard of the Match. Neither had most members of my family. So there was a certain comfort in talking with people equally obsessed by this unusual process and the intense year that would follow. I traded many of my own school's social events for nights out with these medical students. I was a curious outsider to their world, hungry for any information I could find on the possible life that awaited Stephanie and me.

As Match Day approached, I swapped stories at bars and coffee shops with my friends Michele and her boyfriend Ted, both New York Medical College fourth-years, their classmate Rakhi and her husband, Scott. We were bound by uncertainty and anxiety as we waited for the same moment that would determine each of our futures.

Scott, like me, was a foreigner to the medical world and he and I grew close. He sometimes joked with me about the absurdity of this moment when our lives would change. He knew exactly what it would be like, he told me. "It will be a clear and sunny day," he said. "Kind of chilly. All of us will be in a big circle, milling about with anxiety. And then, at the preordained moment, we'll hear the blast of the trumpets. We'll all look toward heaven, and as the clouds softly part, little letters will flutter down from heaven into each applicant's hands, delivered from the hand of God. It will be the perfect moment. Ordained by God," Scott continued, pausing before adding his punch line, "Or Alvin Roth."

His wife, Rakhi, joked about it less. With each passing week approaching Match Day, this woman, considered to be the kindest, friendliest student in the class by her peers, made a valiant effort to cover her angst. Michele also had moments of dread. She grew concerned about her relationship with Ted and wondered whether they would survive the Match.

As I set out to learn about the Match and about residency, their stories became as much a part of my education as Stephanie's own tale.

2

The R.O.A.D. to Happiness

On an early autumn morning, Michele LaFonda made the forty-five-minute trip north from Manhattan's Upper East Side to New York Medical College. The large private medical school in Westchester County, where Michele was a fourth-year student, sat on what felt like isolated land, with a hospital and a juvenile detention facility off in the distance. Still, the college seemed peaceful. A few buildings clustered together to the side of the quiet Sunshine Cottage Road, with the only real disturbances coming from some fearless Canadian geese.

Michele had lived closer to campus at first, but the school gave its students the option of clinical rotations at Manhattan hospitals during their last two years, so she and some friends had fled to the city for the remainder of medical school. She was an extrovert, and Manhattan was a better fit. Endless stretches of coffee shops, restaurants, and bars buzzed just blocks from her apartment. A short subway ride south to the Village on the right night and she could enjoy twenty-cent buffalo wings and two-dollar beers to the tunes of covers from the eighties and nineties. Even with exams and demanding rotations, Michele made time for socializing. In Manhattan she had countless options.

She was twenty-seven years old. Light brown hair fell beyond her shoulders, and nearly perfect white teeth gleamed during body-shaking laughs. She looked stylish. Outside the confines of medicine's world of scrubs and formaldehyde, her keen awareness of fashion often led her to opt for a trendy hat, knit scarf, or big sunglasses. With her first residency interviews starting soon, she wanted to be sure she had the right outfit to make a good impression. So a few weeks earlier, while shopping in a Banana Republic store in Manhattan, she had snapped up an elegant brown pantsuit. It cost three hundred dollars; it seemed the perfect choice.

On days when she needed to be on campus, Michele made the journey north, back to the site of her first two years of training— back to the classrooms, the cafeteria, and the anatomy lab. New York Medical College's anatomy lab was not tucked away in a dark and dreary basement. It sat on the fourth floor atop the Medical Education Center. Natural light streamed in through rows of windows and skylights. Unlike most of her peers, Michele had cut into cadavers even before she first entered that lab. She had never been squeamish, and had worked for a regional tissue bank in Northern California just after college. In the evenings, a pager had summoned her to retrieve skin, heart valves, and corneas from donors who had died within the last twenty-four hours. Sometimes, when she arrived, the bodies were still warm to her touch. But as Michele prepared to remove skin that could be used for burn victims, they became fields of potential skin harvest sites.

Pressing the cold metal of a dermatome against the bodies, she retrieved sheets of skin in uniform and precise thickness. Other times she held scissors with her middle finger and thumb as she had been taught, letting her index finger rest on top as a guide, and removed the clear, dome-shaped corneas from the vacant eyes of the deceased.

On this trip back to the campus, she bypassed the anatomy lab. The hours spent hunched over cadavers, memorizing bones and muscles, arteries and veins, had been only part of the long road to this point in her education that, nearly a decade earlier, began at De Anza Community College in California. Though she had been a strong high school student with a 3.7 grade point average, she never thought about going straight to a four-year college. Her mother had attended a community college, and Michele always assumed she would too. Money was tight. Community college meant she could live at home for free, use a scholarship to pay the tuition, and save money from her afternoon and weekend jobs to prepare for her transfer to the University of California, San Diego. Even at UCSD, she took multiple jobs, working in a lab at the university and as a teacher's aide for children with behavioral problems at a local middle school. She followed her undergraduate degree with a job at a biotech company and nights at the tissue bank while waiting to get into medical school, and finally, with the move to New York Medical College. Now she was almost finished. In six months New York Medical College would declare her a medical doctor, though where she was going and what she would be doing were still up in the air. What remained was the onslaught of discussions about residency interviews, rank lists, and the Match.

Whenever Michele wanted advice, she turned to Dr. Susan

Rachlin, a forty-something-year-old radiologist on faculty. In some ways, Rachlin reminded Michele of her mother—the cool parent, the talkative, confident one who enjoyed chatting with the kids. Rachlin kept a jar filled with candy in the back of her classroom. She gossiped with the ladies. She talked sports with the guys. She loved to tease her students and learn about their lives. And she coached anyone who wanted to pursue a career in radiology. Rachlin encouraged all the New York Medical College fourth-years interested in her field to apply to about sixty hospitals. That number seemed ridiculously large compared to the fifteen or twenty applications Michele's classmates put in for other areas of medicine. But radiology had become one of the more competitive fields. Students needed a savvy guide like Rachlin to help them attain good placements. One year earlier, twenty-six of Rachlin's students matched in radiology residency positions. The year before that, Michele had heard, it was around thirty. Michele hoped to be another one of the professor's success stories.

It was a meeting with Rachlin that pulled Michele back to campus on this day. The fourth-year students had applied to residency programs beginning in September and started receiving interview invitations not long after. Sometime in October, just before the first interviews, Rachlin liked to conduct mock interviews with her students, quizzing them as if they were trying to land residency positions at her radiology department at Westchester County Medical Center.

"Why do you want to be a radiologist?" Rachlin would ask. It seemed like an obvious question, but poorly prepared students came off sounding trite or unconvincing and could find the experience troubling. Every few minutes, Rachlin would provide blunt, practical advice on how to handle the interview better. If students paid attention and heeded her tips, their odds of landing a choice residency could greatly improve.

Even the most peripheral matters—jewelry, body language, and clothing choices—came into consideration for Rachlin's review. Interviewers might appear to be focusing only on medical credentials. But Rachlin, like many others, believed that when students were being interviewed, they were being judged on a much wider and more treacherous set of attributes. Was there anything that might take them away from the time they needed to be at the hospital? Would they be responsible and competent physicians? Did they look sufficiently serious? Over the years, residency lore dictated that, for a woman, this quality could be best conveyed in black, brown, gray, or blue skirts. Rumor had it that Rachlin had already told one female visitor that it might be unwise to go for interviews in a pantsuit. A skirt would be a better choice. That tip had made its way back to Michele. Unlike some students, who might have laughed it off, Michele absorbed it with all the respect accorded to a Supreme Court decision. Now she considered pushing that three-hundred-dollar Banana Republic pantsuit to the back of her closet. Rachlin's dim view of pantsuits wasn't something Michele wanted to fight, although it frustrated her. The younger woman planned to take all of her adviser's suggestions. She trusted Rachlin to help her match into radiology.

There were days when Michele wondered if she was a strong enough candidate. She had only come to consider a career in radiology within the past year—late compared to some of her classmates—even though she grew up with a mother who was an X-ray technician. Her mother's job had shown Michele the world of hospitals and doctors, but it was Michele's love of children that first made her consider medical school. Even at the age of twelve, she told adults that she planned to be a pediatrician. Babysitting for a friend of her mother's, Michele would take a small plastic toilet, place it in the living room, and try to potty-train a little girl named Katie Beth. Other times, she would give Katie Beth a bath. She couldn't imagine a better job than helping children. In medical school, though, each day when Michele came home from her rotation in pediatrics, she relayed stories to her boyfriend, Ted, of how cute the children were or how much fun she had playing with them, rather than showing any excitement about providing them with medical care. Her pediatrics rotation, she realized, confirmed not that this was the type of medicine she wanted to practice, but instead how much she wanted to be a mother.

It was during a radiology elective that her desire to be a doctor really peaked. Here was a field that felt unrestricted. A radiologist could work with a varied group of patients and doctors from many different fields. The scope of the field was all-encompassing. The radiologists she had met possessed an encyclopedic knowledge of the medical world.

But there was one other attractive aspect to radiology that she wasn't sure she'd admit to the interviewers. With the certainty that she wanted children came the importance of a career that allowed her to spend time with and financially support her future family. A radiologist could make more than $300,000 in a year. A radiologist had a more manageable schedule than most doctors. Even a resident's hours were reasonable in this field. There were fewer emergencies, fewer nights at the hospital, and sometimes even nine-to-five days, which were rare in most other residencies. That schedule enabled a radiologist to have a life outside the hospital. Rachlin had three children. She went to their baseball games. She spent time with the kids at home. That's what Michele wanted. Knowing that she'd be thirty-three by the time she finished a radiology residency, she would even consider the possibility of having a child before finishing residency. That's what Rachlin had done.

But Michele knew not to mention any of this on an interview.

The way Michele figured, she had dedicated the last eight or so years, at least, to career goals. Now, as she was hitting her late twenties, she didn't want to neglect the idea of marriage and family. Each time a small child passed her on the street, she smiled. She knew Ted would make a tremendous father. But as she dreamed about a future with Ted, insecurities haunted her.

As a child, Michele's home was rarely a peaceful environment. Her mother and father didn't know how to talk to each other, it seemed, so they just yelled. Michele thought that her father, a Vietnam veteran, tried to run their home the same way he would command troops. He had a quick temper, once telling Michele's brother that the boy would never be allowed to drink milk again after the kid dropped a glass. Michele had learned to turn to her mother, who granted the freedom and independence that a new teenager so often craves.

On her parents' seventeenth anniversary, when Michele was fourteen, she and her younger brother were sent to a friend's house. Home the next morning, Michele walked into her room and saw her bed unmade, the covers crumpled. She searched the house for her mother and asked what happened to her bed. Her mother started crying and explained that she wasn't able to sleep in her own bed that night. So she had climbed into Michele's. Tears streaming down her face, her mother related how Michele's father had left despite pleas to stay, to try to make the marriage work, to go to counseling with her. But he had said he couldn't. And he left that night, on their anniversary.

Michele wept too. She often cried whenever she saw her mother cry, but this time she was also angry. Her father had given up. Her mother had been abandoned. And they would eventually need to move out of their house. There was no question who Michele would stay with. Though her father ended up living just twenty minutes away, Michele often saw him only on holidays.

Thirteen years later, one of Michele's greatest fears was that Ted would wake up one day and decide to leave her. He was a good-looking man with broad shoulders, a little over six feet tall, and had played football at the University of Nebraska before enrolling in New York Medical College. But he was gentle, with a soft smile and soothing tone. Like Michele, he was in his fourth year and about to begin residency interviews. After more than a year of dating, Michele became convinced that she wanted to marry him. But she also sensed his ambivalence. Rank lists were due in just a few months. She begged him to spend some time considering whether they had a future together. She wanted him to decide whether he looked at her as his potential wife or merely as a temporary girlfriend. Would he continue to date her for years and then abandon her if he realized he wanted something different? Michele brought it up again and again during the year leading up to Match Day, hoping that he would give it thought. She'd rather hear bad news from him now, she told him, than in five years.

• • •

Michele told me how Rachlin held a copy of her application in her hands during the mock interview. "So, why do you want to go into radiology?" the doctor asked Michele.

"Um, so when I was little," Michele began, "my mom was, um, an X-ray tech and I used to go to work with her all the time and . . ."

Rachlin let Michele finish. "Do you know you said 'um' about thirty times?" she said.

Despite her corrections, there was a charm to Rachlin's coaching, especially when she smiled. She was to the point, but she was on Michele's side. She told her to rehearse the answer. Get comfortable with your response so you don't feel awkward. And make sure you know how to end it. Try concluding the answer with something like, "And that's why I want to go into radiology," she suggested. And if Michele was ever asked, "Why do you want to come to this program?" she could talk about the size of the program, Rachlin explained. If it was a big program, you wanted a big program; if it was small, you wanted to be in a small program. Of course, one answer that would never fail would be, "I sat down with my adviser and she felt this would be a good program for me." Rachlin said, "If people ever tell me that, I get so excited. Oh, they were talking about me?"

Radiologists are particularly attuned to using visual clues to make a diagnosis, and Rachlin's observations were sharp when she met with her students for the mock interviews. She had a list of suggestions in terms of appearance. For the women, nails should be kept short. Makeup should be conservative. And if Rachlin saw an engagement ring, she offered one more thought: consider taking it off.

She didn't want to push her students to do anything that made them uncomfortable. It was up to them if they wanted to take it off. At the same time, she was protective of her students. She believed it was her job to help them understand how certain clues might be interpreted. Laws prevented interviewers from asking about spouses, partners, or plans to have children. But that didn't mean that some wouldn't try. And it didn't mean that the interviewer wouldn't notice a wedding or engagement ring. For a male student, Rachlin thought a noticed ring was not a concern. A married man might even hint at more stability in a candidate. For a woman, it was more complicated.

Although Rachlin felt that most program directors strived for equality, she also knew that seeing a ring on a woman's finger might subconsciously affect their decisions and lead some people to see a married woman as a potential babymaker. Although the world of medicine had made progress toward gender equality, some residency directors, she worried, might still be influenced by concerns about pregnancies. With a pregnant resident came possible added complications for a residency director and fellow residents. In radiology, there would be concerns about exposing a pregnant woman to radiation. In other specialties the strenuous call schedule raised questions. Would she need more time off than the vacation schedule allowed, and if so, how would the other residents cover for her? No program wanted one of its residents to get pregnant. With a limited number of residents and each resident carrying a large number of patients, if one was absent, the others would have to pick up the slack. Coresidents would feel dumped on. A difficult pregnancy, requiring an extended time away from work, had the potential to alter things within a program. Rachlin wanted to say that it wasn't true, that it was unfair and should be dealt with as a matter of course. Still, she was concerned about how an applicant might be perceived by some people.

She told her students never to lie. If they were asked about relationships, they should be polite and answer whatever they felt comfortable answering. But there was also no need to volunteer information.

Rachlin glanced at the hobbies section of Michele's application. "Oh, you like movies," she said, mimicking the chitchat of a real interview. "What movies have you seen lately?"

"Well," Michele began, "we went to—"

"Who's we?"

Michele froze.

The doctor offered some counsel for the young woman after the misstep. "You're giving them an opportunity to start questioning you about it," she said.

It wasn't that Rachlin was against the idea of having children while being a doctor or a resident. On her desk sat a photograph of her three sons. Family was important to her, and though she described herself as having such a full plate it was probably cracked, she relished her multiple roles: teaching, working as a radiologist in the hospital, being a mother, and being a wife. She appreciated how a career in radiology allowed for a more controlled lifestyle than other specialties.

In talking to her students, Rachlin was speaking in part from her knowledge as a residency director. But she was also influenced by the negative reactions she had received each time she had become pregnant. The first time, pregnant with her son Jordan, she was in her last year of residency in the early 1990s. She had hoped to keep the news quiet for a bit, but told her program director so that she could avoid any radiation that might prove harmful to the pregnancy. She asked that the news be kept in confidence. When she learned that a staff meeting had been called the next day to discuss her pregnancy, Rachlin was furious. She felt betrayed. She felt as if she was no longer a person to them, just a problem.

After she began to show during her second pregnancy, now out of residency and working full-time, a new boss called her in and demanded to know why she hadn't mentioned she was pregnant during her interview. Not that it would have mattered, he quickly added. Finally, when she announced her third pregnancy, a female boss threw down a pencil, cursed, and screamed, "That's it. I will never hire another pair of ovaries to work in this department again." Given her history, Rachlin was protective of her female students and suggested they avoid the subject on their interviews.

As Michele's mock interview was wrapping up, Rachlin brought up attire. She confirmed what Michele had heard from the friend. With the possibility of older, conservative doctors interviewing the candidates, a skirt was still what they would consider business attire for women. It was better to play it safe.

"In three years, I might not say this," Rachlin said. "But for right now, I think it's something you need to do."

After the third or fourth time Michele told me of some counsel she received from Rachlin, I decided to make the trip up to Westchester County to meet her mentor. I joined Rachlin's radiology elective at the medical school just after lunch one afternoon. Students filtered into the classroom chatting and found their way to stations set up around the room to work in groups. There seemed to be an even mix of men and women. Forty years earlier, the classroom would have looked drastically different. Then, less than 7 percent of the country's graduating medical students were women. But by 2005, the national percentage had grown to 47. And at some medical schools, there were now more women than men in the entering classes.

Trailblazers from past generations had broken the gender barrier for these women. Rachlin kept a *New York Times* obituary for one such pioneer—her own professor from medical school, Dr. Lucy Squire—pinned to a bulletin board on the side of her room. But even as I sat in the classroom, nearly three out of four physicians who practiced in the United States were still male. It would take this new generation of doctors to truly change the face of the profession.

I sat by Rachlin in the back of the room. I told her that I was interested in learning how women balanced a demanding career in medicine with family, at an age when many considered having children. I explained that Stephanie, my girlfriend, was planning to match in surgery.

"I'd suggest you get a new girlfriend," Rachlin joked.

I gave her a little laugh and smile. A lot of our friends had responded similarly. "I can't believe Stephanie is going into surgery," or, "you won't see her for seven years, at least," or, "wow, good luck with that."

Rachlin told me that there had been a brief period when she was tempted by a career in surgery. She had been at the start of her fourth year of medical school in Brooklyn, at the school known today as SUNY Downstate and, in preparing for her residency applications, had looked into both surgery and radiology. Radiology was the natural choice, her goal ever since childhood, when she learned about the field from a cousin. She was always visual, able to pick out the hidden picture in a *Highlights* magazine in a matter of seconds. But in medical school, she had also been tempted by the excitement of watching surgeons at work. The operating room captivated her. After drowning in books for the first two years of medical school, the operating room felt action-packed. Her heart raced as she stood there, enthralled. She figured she would apply to residencies in both surgery and radiology and decide later, after the interviews.

The more Rachlin thought about it, though, the more her love of radiology pulled her back and concerns about a surgeon's lifestyle pushed her away. After attending a memorial service for one of the young surgeons from her hospital that fall, her feelings were only confirmed.

By then the surgeon's death had made national news. A cabdriver had entered Rachlin's hospital wearing a blue ski coat and carrying a blue canvas shoulder bag, in which he had hidden a sawed-off shotgun. He walked down a hallway on the building's fourth floor and, through an open office door, fired the gun. The motive was unclear—the cabbie had been a former patient, but not of this doctor—and the young surgeon died in the hospital's operating room an hour later.

At the memorial, Rachlin looked at the doctor's wife. She saw their three young children, all in diapers. Their father did not seem many years out of his surgical residency. He probably had been pushing through those years of residency, Rachlin thought, until he'd be able to enjoy his family. Once he got through, his life was taken. Rachlin realized she had no idea how much time she had to live. So she pulled her surgery applications and decided to stay with radiology, her true passion.

"What many surgical residents will say is, 'I just have to get through residency,'" Rachlin told me. "'Once I get through residency, everything will be okay.' It's almost as if in their mind they're going to toss away seven years of their life. They say, all right, I'm just going to get rid of those. I just have to do it. And I'm sure that's exactly what this young surgeon thought to himself, that I just have to get through this time and then I'll be able to enjoy my family. And once he got through that time, his time was gone.

"It's a very tough life," she continued. "By the same token, we need surgeons. We have to have good surgeons. We have to have well-trained, highly qualified people to do that." She paused. "They don't necessarily have to be your girlfriend," she added, then laughed.

If I were the one pursuing a career in surgery, Rachlin's story would have hit home. Learning from my father's experiences, I knew I wanted to balance career with ample family time and not toss away any years. But I wasn't the one making the decision to become a surgeon. While it seemed unusual for me to hear words of warning about a career in surgery from a medical professor, I was not stunned. Rachlin worked in what medical students deemed a lifestyle-friendly specialty, and she sounded more like a doctor of my generation than of her own.

After socializing with medical students for the past year, I had grown used to hearing about lifestyle specialties. The medical students I knew went into medicine for the same reasons as those in generations past—they wanted to help people; it was a challenging career; it was well respected. But they also valued lifestyle. In deciding what specialty to go into, many medical students spoke of something called the R.O.A.D. to Happiness.

"R.O.A.D." stood for residencies in radiology, ophthalmology, anesthesiology, and dermatology. These specialties usually paid better than a career in family or internal medicine. For students leaving medical school with an average debt of more than $100,000, income was an important consideration. A R.O.A.D. specialty also meant a better ability to have what doctors called a controllable lifestyle. On the R.O.A.D., schedules were more predictable. There were fewer emergencies. Nights spent on call at the hospital were limited. On the R.O.A.D., a doctor could reliably make good on commitments other than work. On the R.O.A.D., becoming a doctor did not mean choosing career over family.

The allure of R.O.A.D. specialties did not go unnoticed. The medical field constantly examines itself. Academic articles in medical journals not only address developments in treatments or discoveries in the research of diseases, but also the practice of medicine itself. Reasons for entering the field, length of career, suicide and divorce rates are all placed under the microscope. Around the time my friends were in medical school, many journal articles picked up on this emerging preference for a balance of work and life.

One article, from *The Journal of the American Medical Association* in 2003, noted that 92 percent of senior medical students viewed general surgeons as not having adequate control over their time. At the same time, the article noted how the Match had seen an increase in the percentage of U.S. students applying to programs in anesthesiology and radiology. These weren't the only specialties seeing a rise. One dermatologist noted that while the number of positions offered in his field had remained about the same for three decades, the number of applicants continued to climb, and the quality of the applicants only improved. Other students and doctors spoke of the E-R.O.A.D. or R.O.A.D.E., adding emergency medicine, with its tendency toward shift work, to the desirable list. All this left leaders in family medicine and general internal medicine concerned that their residency positions would go unfilled and that they would need to take more international medical students to fill the slots. Just two months before the 2006 Match, the American College of Physicians released a report and statement that noted that primary care was "on the verge of collapse," with very few young physicians going into the field.

Articles pointed to a change in priorities from the medical students of the 1980s, who listed lifestyle and personal factors as being the least important in making a career choice. The interesting thing was, despite two defining characteristics of the new generation of medical school graduates—a growth in the number of women and an increase in the desire for specialties with better lifestyles—the studies found that women were no more responsible for this move to a better lifestyle specialty than men. But not all residency programs were as gender balanced as medical schools. In 2005, there were plenty of gender-lopsided residencies. More than 75 percent of residents in obstetrics and gynecology were women, more than 72 percent of surgical residents were men, and more than 70 of pediatric residents were women. Still, men of my generation were looking toward specialties with controllable lifestyles too. Just as Michele had decided on a career in radiology, her boyfriend, Ted, ended up applying in anesthesiology. If you wanted to become a doctor but were not ready to give up every other aspect of your life, there seemed no better path than the R.O.A.D.

One of Ted's two major problems going into his fourth year of medical school had been not knowing what type of doctor he wanted to become. He enjoyed surgery but couldn't stand surgeons. They were all so arrogant, he once told me sheepishly, and he couldn't see himself around people who rarely admitted they were wrong. Also, they seemed to have no lives away from the hospital. Ted, who was twenty-eight years old in the year he would Match, had always enjoyed more than just medical work.

When Ted was a boy, on days when the radio signal had not come in clearly at his family's home in Iowa, his father packed his two sons into a car and drove up to the highest hill he could find just outside their small town in the northwest corner of the state. Lincoln, Nebraska, was a good two hundred miles south, but Cornhusker football was king in these parts of the country, and there was no doubt what Ted's family had on the schedule for Saturdays during football season. From the right spot on that hill, they could tune in a station from Sioux City and cheer on Coach Tom Osborne's boys. A good season meant the Huskers lost only one of their twelve or thirteen games. A bad season meant two, at worst three, losses.

Only about seven hundred families lived in the small town where Ted's father ran a local market. Neither of Ted's parents had attended college, but they had strong work ethics. They stressed education and hard work with their boys, made them wax the store's floors once a week and carry out groceries for the customers. At other times, Ted was sent to help at his uncle's furniture store or his cousin's carpet shop.

It was impossible for Ted—or nearly anyone in the town—to walk from one place to another without being stopped for a chat. Though he looked embarrassed and smiled when I teased him that he was the corn-fed, all-American boy, it was not hard to picture Ted this way. He was a smart, capable man who seemed to have participated in just about every activity in high school—he was quarterback and safety for the football team, played for its basketball and baseball teams, ran for its track team, served as student body president, was a member of the homecoming court, and sang and danced onstage during the school's musical productions. "There was one advantage of the small town and small school," he told me. "You didn't have to be the specialist there."

Still, not every football player from his school was invited by Tom Osborne to walk on to the Nebraska football team. Ted couldn't keep his father quiet when he brought him to Osborne's office for his official visit. Neither Ted nor his father considered any other university when they learned he could play safety for Osborne. And with his 3.9 high school grade point average, Ted found himself enrolled in the University of Nebraska Honors Program, which left his parents beaming.

There was no one moment when Ted decided to become a doctor. That career just seemed to him to play to his strengths. His mother, like Michele's, had been an X-ray technician and occasionally took him to work with her, where he watched the doctors and medical professionals. In school, Ted loved his science classes, and his affection for the sciences continued in college. To balance the demands of an unforgiving football schedule and rigorous premed course load at the university, he scheduled physics labs for the evenings after practice. He studied in the early mornings and again from 8 P.M. to midnight.

But Ted wasn't used to asking for help, and he applied to medical school with no more guidance than the tips he gathered from reading a book he picked out at the local Barnes and Noble. His college grades—a 3.6 GPA—were average for a medical student, his test scores nothing spectacular. The first time he applied, he didn't get in to any medical schools. But he kept an optimistic attitude. He had wanted to take a year off before medical school anyway, he told himself. The second year, when the same thing happened, his anger mounted. After his third year of applications, Ted was bound for New York Medical College.

More than most of his peers, Ted put off making hard decisions. He hated confrontation, couldn't stand to hurt people, and usually went with the maybe-it-will-go-away-if-I-don't-think-about-it option. In the year before the Match, Ted felt pressured not only to decide what area of medicine to apply for, but also to answer Michele's questions about their future.

Between the two issues, deciding his specialty was the easier one. Anesthesiology seemed like a perfect fit, allowing him to work with his hands and to be in the operating room. A career in anesthesiology also permitted him to keep the social life he had grown used to since moving to New York—nights listening to jazz in crowded clubs, and plenty of athletic activities. But even as Ted made up his mind about his career, he couldn't find answers for Michele.

After more than a year of dating, things seemed to be going well, but Ted wasn't prepared to make a lifetime commitment just yet. Perhaps he and Michele would start a life and family together. On one hand, he was constantly touched by her warmth and her kindness, both to him and to strangers. Once, when they were standing outside a club, waiting for their friends, a drunk stranger stumbled to the curb and had trouble moving. Michele stayed there, talking to the woman and comforting her, until an ambulance arrived. But when cornered on the subject, Ted also wondered if, as a mother, she would try too hard to be her children's best friend. He wondered if Michele got away with too much as a teenager. Even though she had always done well in school, he knew she had never been shy about partying with her friends, and that her mother had no problem with it. Still, her behavior had not damaged her education or career.

It drove Michele crazy, but often when Ted spoke to his mother on the phone, he left out updates on Michele or her life. Maybe he viewed Michele as the woman you dated before you got serious, or maybe she really was the one. But Ted didn't see why he needed to think about that now. Both he and Michele wanted to stay in New York, and they talked about how they both planned to rank New York programs in the top three or four spots on their rank lists. It frustrated him that Michele brought up questions about their future. Wasn't this what dating was for, anyway, to figure out if a relationship would last?

Though it had taken him a while to come around, Ted now regularly told Michele he loved her. He just couldn't tell her what he'd want several years from now. And he worried about hurting her if he didn't have the right answers to her questions. So Ted did what he always did. He just avoided the subject.

After the residency interview season started, I asked Ted how often he was questioned about family during his interviews. Not once, he said. Michele, however, mentioned that a few of her visits were tinged in vague, hard-to-prove ways with curiosity about her personal life. Usually questions were straightforward and simply revolved around some aspect of her résumé—"Oh, you went to community college. Tell me about that"—or focused on why she went to medical school or why she wanted to go into radiology. Sometimes they made small talk with her, asking her about football, since she had listed watching the sport under a hobbies section. But on occasion, she was asked if she was single. On one interview, a woman asked her if she was married and had children. Rather than just answer no, Michele launched into her speech, prepared for this very moment.

"Well, a family is something that I'm interested in," she said. "I don't have one now, but I don't feel it would be fair to start a family while I'm in my residency program. It wouldn't be fair to myself. It wouldn't be fair to my children."

Days on the interview trail saw Michele meeting with four or five people, each for about twenty minutes. There was also the standard tour of the facility, and sometimes the opportunity to sit in on a presentation by one of the residents or attending physicians, as the doctors who supervised the residents were called. It was a busy winter for Michele. Not only did she have dozens of interviews for radiology programs, but because the specialty began its training in the second year of residency—unlike surgery, internal medicine, pediatrics, or a number of other fields—Michele also needed to apply to programs solely for her internship year. The same was true for Ted's training in anesthesiology. So both Michele and Ted lined up a set of interviews for preliminary positions for post-graduate-year one and another set of interviews for their specialties, which would cover the remaining three years of residency for an anesthesiologist and four for a radiologist. Between the two of them, they would need to submit four rank lists to the National Resident Matching Program.

As if that wasn't complicated enough, Michele wondered about the couples' match. When she and Ted started dating, Michele had thought that if they didn't ultimately sign up for the couples' match, they would probably break up. It would be a sign of a lack of commitment, she thought. But now she was not so sure. The couples' match was a way to enter the National Residency Matching Program as one unit, creating an "if this then that" list of possibilities that would enable two applicants to end up in residency programs in the same vicinity. Were Ted and Michele to enroll as a couple, their joint rank order list might note that if Ted were to end up at NYU's anesthesiology program, Michele's first choice would be radiology at Westchester County Hospital, her second choice Long Island Jewish, and so on, creating an order of preferred combinations. The couples' match could guarantee that Ted and Michele would end up in the same city, with the opportunity to live together, if that was what they wanted.

"Have you ever thought about couples matching?" she asked him one night in January. They had just finished watching a stranded Tom Hanks in *The Terminal* at Ted's apartment.

Ted seemed surprised. "What do you mean? Wouldn't we have already had to tell them?"

"No," Michele said. A candidate was not designated for the couples' match until the final rank lists were due in late February.

"I didn't know that," Ted said. "I didn't think it was a possibility so I didn't think about it."

Michele told him that she had. She had grown attached to the idea of matching at Westchester Medical, where Rachlin was the radiology program director, and thought about ranking it number one. She knew Ted was debating between Columbia, NYU, and Yale—New Haven didn't seem so far—and if he got any of those, Michele figured they had a shot at being together. But Ted had also interviewed at programs outside the New York area, including ones in Los Angeles, Miami, Houston, Chicago, and Kansas City. They were not his top choices, he told her, and since most people landed somewhere in their top three, he did not think there was much to worry about.

Maybe he was right. Because both she and Ted wanted to stay in the New York area and planned to place local programs at the top of their individual lists, the odds were that a couples' match would not make much difference in their results. But there was a psychological aspect too. Designating the couples' match meant commitment. It also meant taking more control over the fate of the relationship. Michele did not want to give up on the idea. The next time she brought it up, Ted told her he did not want to do anything without knowing how the process worked. So Michele agreed to look it up.

Trying to read the instructions online, though, Michele grew frustrated. The couples' match seemed more complicated by the fact that since residencies for both of their specialties did not include intern year, they each had two lists. The whole process was confusing. She read that each partner of a couple could rank up to thirty different programs before a fee of thirty dollars per additional program popped up, but Michele could not tell if this meant thirty possible combinations or thirty programs each. With all of their possibilities, she wondered if the couples' match would cost a fortune. It seemed it would take a lot of effort. And Ted had yet to say he wanted to do it. Ultimately, Michele stopped pushing. She and Ted decided they would both rank New York programs in their top three spots and see what happened.

• • •

In early February, Michele told me how she went in for one more meeting with Rachlin. This time, it was to discuss the programs she intended to rank. Rachlin looked over the list. Westchester was at the top, followed by Long Island Jewish and nineteen other programs. The first five were all in New York. After Rachlin went through the list, telling Michele her impressions of each program, she stopped.

"Why do you want to be in New York?" Rachlin asked. "Do you have family here?"

"No, I'm from California," Michele said.

"Oh, yes. I should have known that," she said. "So why do you want to stay in New York so badly?"

Michele paused. She remembered what she had been taught about not volunteering any information. But she was not worried about Rachlin judging her.

"Well," Michele said, "my boyfriend's here."

"Did I know you had a boyfriend?" Rachlin asked.

"I don't know."

"How long have you been dating?" Rachlin asked.

"About a year and a half."

"Is it serious?"

Michele certainly felt it was serious. She looked at Ted and saw the man she wanted to spend the rest of her life with. But she still did not know how to answer. "Well, that's kind of what we're trying to figure out," she told Rachlin.

Rachlin asked if they had thought about the couples' match, and Michele explained that with the twenty-one programs she planned to rank, it did not seem as if it would work well. Plus, she explained, outside of his top three programs, they did not have any cities that would overlap. "But his top three choices are NYU, Columbia, and Yale," Michele said.

"He's probably going to get one of those," Rachlin reassured her. "Do you see this relationship going very far?"

"I think I do," Michele said. "But I don't know if he knows."

What Rachlin said next stuck with Michele. The professor explained how she had generally seen two types of relationships between medical students during her years as a teacher. There were those of convenience and those that were going to last, she said. When it came to the Match, couples either broke up or decided to go for it. The Match forced you to make that decision.

"Yeah," Michele said. "I think if this whole Match works the way we want it to, then we'll be together, and if not, then we'll deal with what happens."

The next day, Michele sent Ted an e-mail:

> *Rachlin said something that really got me thinking, you'll hate her for this . . . either we're a couple of convenience that won't make it past med school or we are a couple that is committed to making this relationship work. Do you agree? Or is there grey zone? I guess I want to know where you think we fall, or where you want us to fall. I am sorry, I know you hate talking about feelings, but my rank list isn't as straightforward as yours and I need some help.*

3

The Rank List

Sitting in a room with her husband, Scott, and four other friends from church, Rakhi Barkowski held a white sheet of paper in her hand. This week's scripture was from the Gospel of Mark, and the passage, printed on the handout, dealt with the healing power of forgiveness. It is not the righteous who need help, but the sinners, the passage reminded them. "It is not the healthy who need a doctor, but the sick," it said. Rakhi looked at the page. In three months she would graduate from medical school and officially become a doctor—Dr. Barkowski. Though it didn't reflect her Indian ethnicity as her maiden name had, she had taken Scott's last name when they were married after her first year of medical school.

For much of their marriage, Tuesday night had been Bible Study night. And when Tuesday fell on February 14, as it did this particular week, it meant that the Empire State Building's red glow lit up the sky some sixty blocks south and that men and women crammed into the city's subways and buses with red roses clenched in their hands. It meant that restaurant reservations had been booked weeks in advance, and that on this Valentine's Day, Rakhi and Scott were sitting across from each other in a friend's living room on Manhattan's Upper East Side.

I had asked to join them and I now sat watching Rakhi. She was a petite woman, a little over five feet tall, with dark skin and long black hair. She listened as the conversation around her turned from a discussion on forgiveness and healing to a casual debate over the varying degrees of suffering. She was aware that people tended to consider her a kind, sweet woman, and she tried always to think of others. But today, and for the past few weeks for that matter, she had a hard time not feeling absorbed in her own life.

"Sometimes I think when I open that envelope, if it's not my number one, I feel like I'm going to suffer," she said. She constantly thought about Match Day, now only a month away. Rakhi had sent in her application to internal medicine programs, she had gone on interviews, and just that afternoon, she had entered what the National Residency Matching Program called a rank order list into her computer. In the list, she had noted and ranked her sixteen choices for programs, but she planned to look it over one more time before next week's deadline. At that point, all that would remain would be three weeks of waiting. Although Rakhi had begun the year-long application process in a calm state, with each passing week, that one day in March seemed to occupy more of her thoughts. She woke up to dreams of being handed the envelope, and she found herself analyzing which students in the class had stronger records than her own.

Scott sat on the couch across from her chair. He wore a pressed button-down shirt, having come straight from work. He told Rakhi, as he had many times before, that she shouldn't get worked up if she didn't get her number one choice. A second choice would still be a wonderful opportunity for her. Not getting her number one was no reason to suffer—"That's obviously really stupid," he said, in the blunt manner Rakhi had grown used to. She stayed quiet. She might argue with him in private, but there was no point in fighting here.

Scott knew that Rakhi would continue to worry, so he added another thought to his comment. Suffering was relative, he believed, and no matter why we suffer, "Jesus really feels compassion."

Scott had his own worries, though—ones that he rarely talked about. He usually made a point of pushing what he felt were irrational thoughts out of his mind; no use worrying about something until you know for sure. But, like Rakhi, he was drawing closer to a time when his future seemed up in the air. So when the Bible Study host went around the room to ask if anyone had personal prayer requests before they prayed, Scott spoke first.

"I could start hearing from schools in the next week or so, so I pray for that," he said. After two years of rejections from Ph.D. programs in economics, Scott was making a third attempt. He had moved to New York for Rakhi and taken a job working in a consulting firm that helped prepare expert witness testimony in financial court cases but, despite long hours, he didn't always feel challenged. "So there's that. And there's Rakhi trying to do our rank list, and I pray that we do it the right way," he continued. "It's not that hard, but it's big decisions."

Other voices around the circle slowly spelled out additional specific requests—direction for a couple deciding whether it was the right time to move out of the country; guidance for a friend who was having a difficult time in her career—and then the group bowed their heads as the hostess started the prayer for all of them.

"Dear God, thank you for letting us be here today and worship you," she said. "I thank you for the words you've given us today and that you are compassionate."

Then, after a brief pause, the woman sitting next to Rakhi spoke. "Father," she said, "I lift up Rakhi and Scott tonight as they are near the top of a hill and can't see over it to the beautiful valley beyond."

Rakhi told me how one week later, on the afternoon when her rank order list was due, she sat at the computer in her and Scott's Upper East Side apartment. There wasn't much in the room where they kept the computer—just enough space for a desk, a chair, and sometimes Scott's guitar and amplifier. The bedroom in the apartment was barely large enough to fit their bed. The kitchen made up one side of the living area, and she and Scott had decorated the other side with a few black-and-white photographs from their wedding.

Rakhi fiddled with the keyboard and mouse and began to check her e-mail. She had the rest of the day all planned out. She would try a new recipe for dinner—Chicken Curry in a Hurry—from the Rachael Ray cookbook Scott had given her on her birthday. They would check her rank list one last time before the 9 P.M. deadline, and then they would celebrate. Finally, her list would be in, and the yearlong, anxiety-ridden process known as the Match would be one step closer to completion. All that remained after this night was the wait until Match Day, March 16, when she'd get that envelope.

Landing either of her top two choices—University of California, San Francisco, or Stanford—would allow Rakhi to live near her family for the first time in nine years. Her family had always been important, and she thought nine years was too many to be away. For almost her entire life, she had lived in the San Francisco Bay Area. Rakhi was born in Khandwa, India, where she lived in a house with her mother and fifteen other relatives—aunts, uncles, cousins—and no running water. Her uncle had come to the United States first and earned an M.B.A. at Berkeley, and he had urged Rakhi's father to join him in California. Rakhi's father did, when Rakhi's mother was pregnant with her, and a year later, in 1981, he sent for Rakhi and her mother. She was eleven months old when she moved to the United States and met her father for the first time.

Growing up, Rakhi saw her parents always working hard, juggling various jobs and night classes, rotating schedules so that someone would be home to feed Rakhi and her younger brother, Milan, in the evenings. Often Rakhi was home alone, watching Milan. She felt responsible for her little brother. Though she was not even ten years old on the day of San Francisco's major earthquake in 1989, when the rattling began, Rakhi had grabbed her brother. They ran into the backyard, where they stayed for hours, afraid and alone. Rakhi still felt close to her family, despite being across the country from Milan, a college student at UC-Berkeley, and from her parents, who lived in San Jose.

But though matching at either of her top two choices would put her back in the San Francisco Bay Area, there was a big difference to Rakhi between her number one and any other school. Her dream was to land an internal medicine residency position at UCSF. Its three hospitals had it all—the bread-and-butter cases, as common patient problems were called, and the zebras, those obscure and difficult-to-diagnose cases referred to the nation's major hospitals. And it cared for an underserved population. Rakhi knew that this university had one of the strongest training programs in the country, a program equaled only by those at Harvard and Johns Hopkins. Harvard, Johns Hopkins, and UCSF had all denied her interviews at first. But strong board scores and a telephone call from her dean had helped Rakhi claw her way into an interview at UCSF, convincing the school that it had made a mistake.

Her interview completed, she desperately wanted UCSF to want her. That would prove the program wrong for initially passing her over, and it would mean that she had truly excelled in medicine. She had e-mailed UCSF's internal medicine residency program director at the beginning of the month to let him know that she planned to rank UCSF number one.

> *It is clear to me that UCSF has the most to offer. In particular, UCSF is unmatched among its peers in the quality of medical training, and has a unique combination of compassionate patient care, commitment to the underserved community, pioneering research, and a mission to shape future leaders in the medical community. Additionally, UCSF's location is ideal for me as a Bay Area native. My family lives in the area, and my desire is to return home for residency.*

The response had come the very next day, and Rakhi read it close to a dozen times, looking for any sort of indication of whether they would grant her a spot.

Rakhi—

This is great to hear. You are clearly a terrific candidate.

Did that mean they were going to put her high enough on their list that she actually had a shot at matching with them? Or was this a canned answer? Were they just being nice, or did they really want her there? Rakhi hated how little understanding she had of this process; how it wasn't as simple and straightforward as acceptances and rejections.

Now, as she looked at her in-box on her computer, a new e-mail appeared on the screen. It was forwarded from Scott, who was at work, with the subject heading "re: graduate application." She opened the message and scrolled down, her eyes catching an e-mail address on the original note ending in "ucla.edu." After all of his rejections over the past two years, Rakhi thought he didn't have a strong chance of getting an acceptance from UCLA. As she read Scott's message, she realized that the graduate department had responded to an inquiry he had sent earlier in the week and was notifying him that, in a few weeks, he would receive acceptance to its program. She was thrilled. Her cell phone rang just as she finished reading the e-mail.

"Hey!" Rakhi called out.

"I feel like this is great news," Scott said. He sounded more enthusiastic than he had all week.

"It *is* great," Rakhi said. "Maybe we should consider moving UCLA," she added, referring to its number three spot on her list, due in just a few hours.

"Yeah, I think so," Scott said.

As they got off the phone and Rakhi reached for a book, a

strange feeling washed over her. Had Scott really gotten in to UCLA? She had never seriously considered what she would do if he was accepted there, and now she felt the pain of replacing Stanford with UCLA as number two on her list. She had tried to get Scott's input about her list before, but he had never pushed any one location. Now she wondered why they had waited so long to talk about her list. She felt a little dizzy.

The phone rang again. This time it was Rakhi's friend Sarah.

"Scott just put me in a tailspin," Rakhi said. "He's pretty much in at UCLA. I need to put it number two on my list. I don't know if I can do it."

Like Rakhi, Sarah was a fourth-year medical student at New York Medical College, also applying to residency programs. "You need to tell him to come home and talk about it," she said. "You both need to be happy with your decision."

There was some urgency in Sarah's voice and, for Rakhi, that was the permission she needed to panic.

"Sarah," she asked, "what if he wants me to move it to number one?"

"You need to call him and tell him to come home," Sarah said.

Rakhi hung up the phone. It was just a few minutes before 6 P.M., only three hours until the computer would stop allowing applicants to make changes to their rank lists. She decided to send Scott an e-mail instead of calling him at work. She knew he had a lot of work to do, but she asked him to come home by seven that evening. *We really need to hash this out face-to-face,* she thought, *because my number two location is most likely where I'm going to end up. We need to figure this out.*

She hit SEND on the e-mail and sat for a moment. She needed to do something, to be around people. She needed to feel the cold air. She decided to run to her favorite fruit and vegetable stand about a block away—they had the best oranges and apples, broccoli and tomatoes. She grabbed her jacket and raced out the door of her apartment. The sky was already growing dark, and Rakhi wondered if the stand would be closed. All she could think was, *I waited too long. I waited too long!*

The hills of Westwood, California, and the rows of warm red bricks of UCLA's Powell Library and Royce Hall were hardly difficult for Rakhi to imagine. The campus had been the setting for two of the more important changes in her life. It was as an undergraduate at UCLA that Rakhi first made the decision to become a physician, and it was on the same campus that she and Scott had met.

When Rakhi was young, there were two things that her parents had made clear that they wanted for their daughter: she should become a doctor and she should marry an Indian man. As a child, Rakhi had spent years pushing back on the idea of becoming a doctor. When her father mentioned this dream of his for her, she would turn to him and say, "No way. That's the last thing I want to do. I don't want to be a doctor. All Indians are doctors!"

Rakhi had wanted to become a firefighter at one point, and later, when she discovered her love of science, a physicist. It wasn't until midway through college, after realizing how much she loved her physical science classes, that she took an internship at the Santa Monica Medical Center, where she shadowed doctors. Even so, she didn't tell her parents at first, for fear they would get their hopes up. She found herself enthralled when talking to patients, listening to their stories, and she developed a deep respect for the doctors who seemed able to put patients at ease during their most vulnerable moments. It made Rakhi feel good to be there, as if she had a purpose.

She wanted to heal the sick and care for the overlooked. The doctors she would remember from medical school were the ones who sat by patients' bedsides and touched patients' hands as they spoke to them, or the one who helped a dying patient finally go home, after the patient had tried to request this in a foreign tongue.

Though Rakhi had often fought with her parents about becoming a doctor, she never broached the other topic: marrying a non-Indian. When she started going to meetings for the campus's University Presbyterian Church along with its affiliated fraternity, she looked around and the only men she saw were white. *This is perfect,* Rakhi thought, knowing that she wouldn't date any of them. *It won't interfere with school.*

Scott was one of the men at the meetings, and Rakhi grew intrigued as she got to know him as a friend. Sometimes he would forgo traditional politeness in order to speak his mind, and she appreciated this quality. And he was kind—he'd stop by her apartment and offer to walk her to the library, where they could both study. But he also had an edge to his personality that she liked. Whereas her roommates sometimes perceived a callous man, Rakhi saw someone who was honest with her and forced her to face tough questions. "Do you really want to become a doctor?" Scott once asked her with one roommate in earshot. "Why don't you become a teacher? Wouldn't it just be easier?"

But most of all, he seemed persistent. As Scott got to know Rakhi, he wasn't afraid to let her know he was interested. "I think you're cute, you're funny, you're sweet, and you laugh at my jokes," he told her. One night, they went out for pizza at Don Antonio's, and Scott reached for the bill.

"It's not that kind of date," Rakhi said. She knew they should just stay friends, but he seemed so determined.

"Please, Rakhi," Scott pleaded. "Let me do this."

He paid for their dinner, and they walked down Westwood Boulevard to the movie theater to take in a showing of *Scream*. When he walked her back to her apartment, Scott leaned in and gave her a high five.

About four months into their relationship, Rakhi decided Scott was worth the battle that was likely to ensue with her parents. But before she called to tell them about him, they called her. Like many of her relatives, Rakhi's parents had had an arranged marriage. Now Rakhi's mother was on the phone to tell her that Rakhi's picture had been circulating among some of their family friends. A family from Philadelphia had contacted them to express interest.

Rakhi bit her lip for a moment. She sat in front of the television in her Westwood apartment, the phone pressed to her ear. "I have something to tell you," she said. "I have somebody here. And his name is Scott."

Rakhi figured the name would be all her mother needed to hear to know that her boyfriend wasn't Indian.

"How long have you been going out?" her mother asked.

"Don't worry. I'm not rushing things," Rakhi said.

There was an unnerving silence on the other end of the telephone. Usually Rakhi's mother screamed when angry. But this day, she stayed quiet. And though Rakhi later found out that her parents had trouble sleeping that night, neither Rakhi's mother nor her father said anything more on the subject until they met Scott a few weeks later and told Rakhi, "He seemed nice."

Rakhi had asked Scott to open her MCAT scores the second time she took the test. The first time, she had not scored as high as she had hoped and knew her choices of medical schools would be limited. She could not bear the sight of it again. They sat on the balcony of her apartment together, facing each other, and Rakhi handed Scott the envelope. She had watched his face tense as he read the letter to himself. "Oh, Rakhi," he said, and handed it to her. It was the exact same score. She wept and curled up in his arms.

By the time Rakhi reached the corner of Eighty-first and York, the fruit and vegetable stand was nearly empty. She turned in the other direction. She tried to calm herself. She would just buy what she needed for the night's dinner. She ran to the D'Agostino supermarket to look for curry paste. Inside, she searched the aisles. She rarely shopped at this market, and she felt lost.

"Do you have curry?" she asked an employee.

"Curry?" he replied, looking confused.

She turned to another employee who also couldn't give her an answer. "Somebody ought to know if you have curry," Rakhi said. "Somebody ought to know!" She never behaved this way. She thought of herself as someone who never inconvenienced anybody.

"Somebody, can you help me?" she cried out.

When Scott called at 6:30 P.M., Rakhi was in another market, this one on Seventy-ninth Street and First Avenue, still desperately looking for curry paste. She hurried down the aisles, her eyes darting from side to side.

"I'm on my way home," Scott said. He breathed heavily and sounded like he was moving quickly from the office to the subway station. "I can't believe it. I can't believe I'm going to grad school."

Rakhi's stomach dropped. She heard him spout all the wonderful things about UCLA, but she couldn't digest his words.

"I love you," she said, right before they hung up.

In the market, Rakhi gave up and settled on hot Szechuan sauce instead of the curry paste. *Fine,* she thought. *I'll move UCLA up to number two. I'm sure that's where I'll end up.* Putting UCLA number two would probably mean more years away from her family. But she decided it was great news. She thought it would be stupid not to do this for Scott's career.

There were the things Scott wanted to do in life, and the things he felt he should do. He wanted to listen to music—to rock, classical, modern, punk, to Led Zeppelin, Pearl Jam, and Weezer. He wanted to sit and play his guitar for hours. He wanted to take a pen and a notebook and write lyrics, then test them out, maybe even record them onto his computer. He wanted to let the artist inside come out for a romp. With his short, spiky hair and a small tuft on his chin that served as a goatee, Scott looked as if he could fit into a California garage band. But his nature also reminded him of expectations and duty. He wanted to be responsible. He wanted to have a stable job and support his family, which consisted only of him and Rakhi, though the way she talked sometimes, he wondered if she would be pushing for them to add one more to their party in a few years.

Scott was committed to Rakhi. The fact that she was his wife was reason enough, he deemed, to love her always, to provide for her, and, when he thought he knew what was best for the two of them, yes, to argue with her. Still, even when they fought, Scott almost never yelled.

Scott had grown up in Southern California, inland of Huntington Beach, in a middle-class neighborhood just off the 405 Freeway, with his mother, a school nurse, and his father, a police officer, along with two siblings. He had worked his way through high school as a bagger at Albertson's grocery store, then stayed on as a clerk and worked at the video counter to pay his way through Orange Coast College until he transferred to UCLA.

When he moved fifty minutes north to Westwood, Scott left his guitar behind for fear it would distract him. In college, he found he enjoyed economics classes and, after graduating, took a job in a consulting agency, recommended by one of his economics professors. The firm worked in litigation consulting, dealing with expert witness testimonies and providing economic analysis for legal teams. He had been at the job for a year when Rakhi decided on New York Medical College.

During Rakhi's first year of medical school, while she was in New York and he continued working in Los Angeles, Scott sent her a paper ring sizer in the mail. A few weeks later, he met her at Penn Station in New York, carrying his guitar.

"Let's go to dinner as long as we're down here," he said, standing with Rakhi in Midtown. They went to a small Spanish restaurant, though Rakhi, nervous, had trouble eating. After he paid the bill, Scott took her to Central Park, where a horse-drawn carriage was waiting for them. Scott sat opposite Rakhi in the carriage and told her he wanted to play her a new song he had written:

You hold me closer
I can hear your voice
I know you love me
I see your smile
And I know I'm home

Scott got down on one knee. "I have something to ask you," he said.

"Oh, my gosh, I knew it!" Rakhi said.

"Will you marry me and be my wife?"

"Yes," Rakhi said. "Yes, I will."

The two were married during the summer after Rakhi's first year of medical school, and they moved into an apartment in Tarrytown, New York. Scott had given up his job in Los Angeles and, for the next few months in New York, he spent every day on the computer, searching for work. He checked listings on Monster.com and the *New York Times* Web site. He e-mailed former colleagues to see if anyone had any connections or knew of any openings. He applied to anything he could find at the Manhattan litigation and economic consulting firms: LECG, NERA, and Cornerstone Research, among others.

With each passing month, Scott lost a little bit of his confidence and grew a little quieter. Rakhi rarely saw him smile, and when he played his guitar, his repertoire seemed to include only melancholy songs. To save money, he rarely turned on the heat, opting for layers and slippers to keep warm.

Rakhi spent hours at the school library. She regularly reviewed her class notes, and while studying, she wrote more notes in the margins to remind herself of the important points. When she came home from a long day, she would sometimes find Scott had gone on a run, trying to deal with the stress. While Rakhi was on her way to being named to the school's Alpha Omega Alpha chapter, the medical honor society, Scott had lost weight and his face had grown thin.

It was a difficult time for Scott, and not just because he always strived for excellence and now he couldn't find work. He wanted to provide for Rakhi. He hated how her friends thought they were poor because she wouldn't buy food when she went out with them. "Buy food!" Scott scolded her. "It's okay!" He couldn't stand for her friends to think he wasn't taking care of her.

But also, while Rakhi excelled and Scott was at home searching Web sites, she had formed a new group of friends who either frequented dance clubs or bars, or talked only of medicine. Scott enjoyed neither. Though he rarely admitted it, the move had been a big sacrifice.

Six months after he began his job search, Scott took a position with CRA International, an economics consulting firm in Manhattan, for less pay than he was earning in Los Angeles, and at a lower position. The work was fine, and he was able to support his family, but Scott still wasn't satisfied with his career.

When he stopped and thought about it, he wondered if going to medical school was a much less risky path than a lot of other fields. Sure, it was hard work, but there was also an amount of certainty and job security. But if Rakhi really did want to work in clinics, as she sometimes said, and if she wanted to take time off to have children, he wondered whether it was a smart investment for her to be the one going through years and years of school.

Scott debated his own future. He believed that a graduate

degree was almost mandatory to get ahead in any job today. He could go to business school for an M.B.A., or he could do something he was more interested in—something he had been thinking about ever since those economics classes at UCLA—and apply to Ph.D. programs in economics. It seemed practical. He could teach or work for a consulting firm at a higher level. Unlike his current job, graduate school also seemed thrilling. It would be like an art form, with room for creativity and recognition. He let his mind wander, contemplating the various fields he could study, such as labor economics or behavioral economics. Even the algorithm behind the Match, designed by the Harvard economist, intrigued him.

Still, Scott applied only to schools close enough to let him continue living with his wife. Columbia, Yale, Princeton, and NYU all sent back rejections. A year later, he added a few more schools—and still had no luck. By the third time around, knowing Rakhi wanted to return to California for her residency, he applied to half a dozen Ph.D. programs in the state, guarding himself, not admitting to many people that this was a big deal to him. On the Monday night of the week Rakhi's rank list was due, he e-mailed each of the programs, explaining his unique situation. He asked if they could possibly let him know early if they planned to accept him, so he and Rakhi could have this information as they ranked her potential programs.

When she saw him, Rakhi gave Scott a hug. She congratulated him on the great news from UCLA and told him how proud she felt. As she started to put away the groceries in the kitchen, Scott sat on the couch. He asked her to stop what she was doing and come sit next to him.

"Do we have to sit?" Rakhi asked nervously. She didn't want to hear what he was about to ask. "Can't I talk to you from the kitchen?"

Scott made his request again. Rakhi walked over and sat by his side.

"So what do you want to talk about?" she asked.

"The list."

"Yeah, I've been thinking," Rakhi said. "I think I'd be comfortable moving UCLA to number two."

Scott said that was terrific. He told her he was really glad to hear that. Reaching over and touching her hand, he asked, "But have you considered moving it to number one?"

Rakhi felt a sting, and her face flinched. "No!" she said.

Scott looked at her intently. "I can't believe you never even thought about it."

"I can't believe you are even asking me," Rakhi replied.

Scott talked more about how UCLA made so much sense for both of them, for them as a couple, but Rakhi couldn't hear his words. She thought about UCSF, her dream, and she started to cry. The clock read 7:15 P.M. Less than two hours remained before the deadline.

"I don't think I have enough time to let it go," she muttered. "I need time to let it go. I've had my heart set on this and now you're asking me to give it up?"

There was a certain amount of doubt in Scott's mind, and he hesitated, wondering how hard to push Rakhi. But he believed he had to hold some level of leadership in the marriage, some responsibility for making the hard decisions, and he thought, given the new information they had received today, they needed to change her rankings. It was the best case for them as a unit, he believed, for her to put UCLA number one.

Rakhi sat there, crying, listening to Scott repeat how much sense it made. She knew her UCLA interview had gone well. If she put it number one, she had little chance of going anywhere else.

Rakhi shot up. With only an hour and a half left before the deadline, she realized that all the procrastinators would be finalizing their lists. She needed to get back on the computer before the system crashed. At least she should move UCLA up to number two now, while they were talking this through.

Rakhi's fingers flew across the keyboard, and she made the change quickly. Then she turned back to Scott. For years she had been striving in medical school, always pushing herself to do more than was expected, knowing that UCSF was her ultimate goal, the ultimate reward, should she get it. Now he was asking her to change this?

"I've been working for this my whole life," she said. "I've worked really hard. It's been my dream. And now you want me to give that up?"

Scott asked her to try to talk about it rationally, to keep emotions out of the way. He was growing frustrated. He told her he was not going to feel bad for her.

"Are you going to resent me if I don't change it?" Rakhi asked.

"I quite possibly might," Scott said.

The words felt like a dagger to Rakhi. It was a little past 8 P.M., and time was running out. "I need to talk to somebody," she said. She wanted to call their friend, a doctor, from the

Bible Study group. Scott thought that was a fine idea. The two of them sat together, just a few feet from the computer, and Scott held Rakhi's hand as she spoke into the phone.

"I love Scott and I want him to be happy," Rakhi said, after explaining the situation. "I'm scared I'm going to make a poor decision. I don't think I have the capacity to make this decision in half an hour."

Their friend told Rakhi that sometimes things seem bigger than they really are. He didn't know what to tell her except that the decisions we make impact our spouses, and he imagined Scott had made some sacrifices for her by moving to New York.

"Yes, he has," Rakhi said.

The friend continued that UCLA was a strong institution, and working there wouldn't be the end of the world. That being said, he told Rakhi that nobody would fault her if she kept UCSF as her top choice. He knew it was her dream. All he could say was that he'd be praying for her. "God be with you both."

Rakhi had never felt so confused in her life. *If only I had one more night,* she thought. The clock now said 8:30—only half an hour remained before the deadline. Rakhi felt as if she could not breathe, gasping between crying convulsions. She reached for a notecard on which she had scribbled her I.D. and password for the computer system. She handed it to Scott and told him that she couldn't physically do it. He needed to make the change and move UCSF down to number two. She wasn't ready to let it go.

"All right," Scott said. Rakhi watched him from the doorway of their small study. He seemed a stranger to her at that moment. He looked like a man who had pushed away all emotion.

She saw him click some keys, hit SUBMIT, and the screen switched to the confirmation page. Rakhi ran into the living room and threw herself on the couch.

It's gone, she thought. *I can't believe it's gone. There's no hope for it now. I have no hope.* She would never even know if UCSF had wanted her. She would never know if she had been a strong enough candidate.

Scott stayed in front of the computer. He didn't look up. He stared straight ahead at the screen.

Rakhi ran back to the room with the computer. "Change it back," she said. She was frantic. "Change it back!"

"Come on, Rakhi," Scott pleaded. "Please don't make me the bad guy." He begged her to stop crying. He told her it would pass.

"I can't," Rakhi sobbed. "I'm not ready to let it pass." She looked at the clock. It was 8:48 P.M.

Scott's face dropped. "Fine," he said, defeated. "I'll change it back." He reentered the password, put UCSF back into Rakhi's first-choice slot, and moved UCLA back down to number two.

Rakhi relaxed. The tears stopped and her breath slowly came back to her. "Wait," she said. "What if I *do* get in? I'll hate myself forever."

"No, you won't," Scott said. "You'll be happy."

This whole time, UCSF had not seemed real to Rakhi. She didn't fully expect to match there, she just didn't want to give up hope. Now, for the first time, she realized that if she got what she wanted, Scott would have to give up graduate school.

"Oh, my gosh," Rakhi said. "If I *do* get in, then you're pretty much not going to grad school?"

"Yeah," Scott said.

Eight minutes remained before the deadline. Rakhi felt calmer now. She told Scott to change it back. She wanted him to put UCLA number one and UCSF number two on her list. "Just do it," she said. "I didn't realize I would jeopardize your whole future." She told Scott that she was going to leave the room. She would walk to the bathroom so that she wouldn't have to watch, but she felt this was the right thing to do.

In the bathroom, Rakhi stared at the mirror and saw her face, swollen from crying. Her eyes looked bloodshot. She and Scott should have had a contingency plan for every possibility, she thought, so no decision would have to be rushed. She turned on the faucet and splashed water over her eyes. *I'm going to UCLA,* she told herself. *I'm going to UCLA and I'll be happy there.* She opened the bathroom door and walked back toward Scott.

"So? Is it done?"

Scott looked at her. "I didn't do it."

"Scott, you're crazy!" Rakhi shouted. "Do it, do it!" The clock said 9 P.M.

"Really?"

"Yes, do it!" she said.

Scott fumbled with the keyboard for a moment, but the computer wouldn't let him log back in. The deadline had passed.

"Oh!" Rakhi cried out. She ran over, sobbing. Scott wrapped his arms around her. "Don't stop loving me," she said. "I'm so sorry."

"Don't be silly," Scott said. He held her there, silent, while she continued to sob.

4

Match Day

Black Monday arrived three weeks later. For most medical students, the opening act to the most anticipated week of the year was simply a matter of hurry up and wait. At noon Eastern time that day, March 13, 2006, students rushed to computers to learn whether or not the Match had paired them with a position. For the overwhelming majority of fourth-years at U.S. medical schools, more than nine out of ten, the answer was yes. They logged on to a Web site, read a one-sentence message noting, "Congratulations, you have matched!" and were forced to wait the seventy-two remaining hours until Match Day for the details. Still, the threat of not matching was enough to make even the most confident candidate's heart race.

Stephanie had lost track of the time. When she realized I was asking if she had checked her status, her voice picked up speed. She told me she would find a computer and call me right back. A few minutes later, my phone rang. Yes, she said. She had matched.

Professor Rachlin had wanted her radiology elective students to lose track of the time that morning as well. The professor promised to keep her students busy to make the morning less painful. When she finally broke for lunch, students raced down the hall and around the corner to the computer lab. There, Rakhi and Ted both learned that they too had matched. Then Ted sent Michele a text message to her phone to make sure everything had gone favorably for her as well.

Even though the odds of receiving a bad message on Black Monday were slim, the wrong note—"We are sorry, you did not match to any position"—would begin a miserable period known as the Scramble. Twenty-four hours after receiving the rejection, a student needed to return to the computer and download a newly posted list of residency programs with unfilled positions. Just as there were candidates who had been spit out of the machine without a match, there were residency programs that remained unfilled. Pickings were slim for the more popular specialties that were already limited in numbers, such as dermatology, orthopedic surgery, or radiology. But if a student was willing to consider a new specialty or maybe just a part of the country that he or she had deemed unacceptable a few days earlier, the odds of finding a position were still favorable, with more residency slots than U.S. medical graduates.

Immediately after downloading the list, the students worked the phones. Some enlisted the help of friends or the staff at the dean's office of their medical schools. They spoke with residency programs and faxed or e-mailed applications, transcripts, deans' letters of recommendation, or whatever other documents the programs wanted to see. Mentors and professors might speak with programs on an applicant's behalf. Telephone interviews followed. And sometime during this frantic period, a program would offer the student a position that, in all likelihood, he or she would accept. In this regard, the Scramble was an awkward holdover from the angst-producing process that led to the inception of the Match.

Michele had seemed nervous about the odds of becoming a radiologist when she first applied to residencies. But by the time she received her twentieth interview request, she began to believe the numbers were in her favor. Still, she needed confirmation. She wanted to view the Black Monday results from the confines of her apartment rather than at the hospital's computers, surrounded by anxious classmates. Match Day would be a public event. For Michele, it would also be about what was in Ted's envelope. This day, though, was a chance to have a moment of privacy. If something went dreadfully wrong, she would be in the comfort of her home. And if things went as expected, she could take a deep breath and know that there was at least some certainty in her future: she would definitely be a radiologist.

That morning, Michele and four of her classmates sat listening to an elderly doctor tell stories of the day he did not match. She was on a student rotation at the New York Eye and Ear Infirmary. Her second-year resident, knowing the significance of the day, had mentioned that the students could leave whenever they wanted. But a gray-haired physician, who had happened upon them in the halls, felt it an appropriate time to reminisce. Reluctantly, they pulled up chairs in a small conference room. Michele listened for the first few minutes as he spoke of how he had applied to five programs in ophthalmology and did not match into any of them. He was greatly disappointed but, in the end, things turned out for the best, he said. That's how he started working in Ear, Nose, and Throat. Michele checked her watch.

By 12:05, the storytelling was finished. The five students went upstairs to a room with computers. Michele watched two classmates log on and learn of their success. But by the time the third student tried, the National Resident Matching Program's Web site refused to come up, most likely overloaded from the deluge of students all checking their match status at that very moment. After several more unsuccessful attempts, a few of Michele's classmates decided to catch a bus and check from their apartments. Michele agreed to go too, anxious to get to the laptop in her bedroom.

The M15 Limited was an express, shooting up First Avenue from Fourteenth Street to the Upper East Side, where they all lived in the same apartment building. The ride usually took about thirty minutes. Odds were the Web site would be accessible again by the time they got off. Still, that suddenly felt too long for one of Michele's classmates. He desperately wanted an orthopedic surgery position and could not wait to know. He called his family, gave them his password, and asked that they call back with any news. Not long after, his cell phone rang. He jumped up and moved three rows forward. Michele strained to see his face and gauge a reaction, but his back was to her. The other classmates thought it did not look good. They saw him raise a hand to his face. By Thirtieth Street, he returned and sat down next to Michele.

"I didn't get it," he said,

The bus stopped at a red light. "I'm really sorry," she told him.

"You know what," he said, "I'm going to take a cab home." He stepped out the doors and disappeared from sight. The bus continued up First Avenue.

When it reached Ninety-sixth Street, Michele got out. Inside her apartment, she ran to her room and grabbed the laptop. After a few seconds, she saw that the computer could not pick up a wireless signal. That happened sometimes, but now was not a moment of patience for Michele. Then the phone rang. Michele only half listened as her friend spoke on the other end of the line, something about not remembering her password, not being able to log on to see if she had matched. Michele passed the phone to a roommate. She was not prepared to deal with this now. She went to another bedroom in the apartment to try a different computer. Thankfully, the Internet connection here worked. She entered her user name. She entered her password. The screen changed. And there was the message. "Congratulations, you have matched!"

Scott and I talked frequently as we waited for Match Day. One day, I sent him a quick e-mail to see if he was planning to take Thursday off work to go to New York Medical College's Match Day gathering. I mentioned that I was deciding if I would fly to California to be with Stephanie.

"Of course I'm taking off!" he wrote me back. "I can't believe you even had to ask. This is the culmination of years of work on Rakhi's part, not to mention sacrifice on the part of both of us, and the singular determining factor of both of our futures. How could I not be there? Let her go and face that alone? I'd quit my job to be with her if I had to." Then he made sure I was going to be with Stephanie.

"If you are at all serious about Stephanie, then you have to be with her," he wrote.

Some of Rakhi's classmates could be turned off by Scott's

direct manner, especially as compared to Rakhi's soft and friendly nature, but I appreciated the e-mail. The truth was, Scott treasured his marriage. At one point, Rakhi asked him what he thought of a long-distance marriage for part of the year if she matched in San Francisco. He told her no. If she matched in San Francisco, he would find a job instead of attending graduate school and being apart. In the weeks after they submitted the rank list, he reminded Rakhi how proud he was of her and told her, "I want you to be happy on Match Day, whatever happens." What Rakhi wanted was for Thursday to come and go so that the panic would subside and she could finally get excited about the verdict, no matter what it said.

On Wednesday night she spoke both to Scott's parents and to her own on the telephone. Her mother mentioned feeling nervous all day. "Just come back to California. That's all I want," she told Rakhi. "We're so scared."

As Rakhi went to bed Wednesday night, the last thing she heard was Scott's voice. Her eyes were closed when he climbed into bed. "Dear Lord," she heard him say, "I pray that you'll just give us peace with whatever decision has already been made. And I pray for a good night's sleep." With that, Rakhi drifted off.

The alarm on my cell phone rang at 6:30 on Thursday morning. I swatted it off, then held still. Silence greeted me instead of New York's daily symphony of honks and truck rumblings. Outside the window, a thick fog dripped over the hills and onto San Francisco Bay. I had flown back to California the day before, and Stephanie and I spent the night at her parents' home. The house was hidden in the hills south of the city. We would need about thirty minutes to get to the medical school for the Match

Day celebration. The drive, a curvy route along Interstate 280, was one of the parts of California I missed most. From the southern end of the peninsula up to San Francisco, the twists and turns of the highway ran along rolling foothills and reservoir waters. It brought sights of cattle and horses, lush greens in the winter and dusty hillsides in the summer. To the east, the bay widened. To the north, the city waited.

I desperately wanted to live in California. Stephanie did too. She dreamed of staying close to her family. Stanford and UCSF were at the top of her list, though she was tempted by Harvard's Massachusetts General Hospital and its renowned surgery program. The week before Stephanie's rank list was due, the Massachusetts General residency director had left a phone message telling her how well she would fit into the hospital's program. Other hospitals also called or e-mailed.

Another hospital's residency director left two messages on the same day, making me wonder if he had called so many candidates he could not keep them straight: "Hi, Stephanie," that director said on the first message. "We had our faculty rank list last evening. And things went well for you." His next message was more specific. "Hi, Stephanie. Please give me a call. I'd love to chat with you. The short answer version is, if you want to come here, you probably will. But I also want to learn from you if there's any other question about our program and stuff like that."

The phone calls were within the National Resident Matching Program's rules. According to the agreement that all Match participants signed, applicants and programs could "express a high degree of interest in each other and try to encourage future ranking decisions in their favor," but were not allowed to "solicit statements implying a commitment." That meant a dance around the room, with some residency directors trying to learn how much you liked their program.

While Stephanie grew excited with each phone call, she also knew enough to be cautious. We had heard rumors about candidates interpreting messages as guarantees, only to find they did not match at these locations. Nothing prevented a residency program from implying more spots to students than there were positions available, with the hope of firming up chances of landing the second-choice candidates, should the first tier match elsewhere. Still, interest from Harvard's Massachusetts General Hospital made Stephanie question whether it was a mistake not to rank the prestigious program higher on her list. Not long after she got the message, she called to tell me she had moved it up to third.

Logically, a rank list should be no different than the order a student would list if sitting down with acceptance letters from every program he or she interviewed at and ordering them by preference. But I wondered if this was not always the case. Subconsciously, people might be more interested in a program if they knew they had been accepted. I suspected this was why some residency directors made telephone calls. If you knew a program thought fondly of you, perhaps you would rank it higher. Even though Stephanie favored the Bay Area, the fact that Harvard now expressed interest threw her off.

I had lived in Boston once before, leaving Stephanie alone for her senior year of college while I took a newspaper job back East. Our relationship somehow survived, and I had moved back to California after a year, eager to be with her again. But again I found myself away from what I considered home when I left for graduate school. Now I longed for California and wondered if I would be miserable going back to Boston for seven years—away from my family and my friends. With Stephanie in one of the nation's most traditional surgical programs, I feared it would all but guarantee that I would never see her. Would that really feel like home? I tried to have faith that Stephanie would get one of her top two choices.

As we drove toward her medical school, a potted orchid balanced delicately on the floor of the car's backseat. Stephanie wanted to drop it off for her adviser as a thank-you before the ceremonies. At times during medical school, Stephanie would call me and tell me how much she wanted to be like this doctor, a woman she found both intimidating and awe-inspiring. The doctor was one of only a handful of female surgery chairs in the country, and a pioneering liver transplant surgeon. Like her adviser, Stephanie found the liver fascinating. The organ could regenerate from as little as 25 percent to its entire size, she told me one evening. During a medical school rotation on transplant surgery, Stephanie had traveled with the UCSF transplant team to retrieve livers from deceased donors. She had not minded the last-minute calls in the middle of the night or the long hours— usually anywhere between six and ten—spent on her feet during a transplant. With the first incision, Stephanie was entranced by the operation—every cut and each stitch. Time passed without notice. At home, she often daydreamed about becoming a transplant surgeon. It thrilled her, and a residency at UCSF under her adviser would be a winning lotto ticket.

But a surgeon's life was difficult enough. It involved five years of long hours and overnight calls plus, at all the hospitals Stephanie had applied to, two research years for a total of seven years. Then there was the possibility of another one, two, or three years of fellowship if she wanted to specialize. For a transplant surgeon, the lifestyle never got better. Unlike some surgeries, most transplants in the U.S. could not be scheduled in advance. There was no waiting until the morning. Delays in transplanting a harvested liver could lead to a higher risk of organ failure. Stephanie wondered if she would be able to deal with a life that involved frequently leaving her family in the middle of the night, just as her mother had once predicted.

Once Stephanie called me up to describe a photograph she had seen while meeting with her adviser's husband, also a renowned surgeon at her school. Stephanie was there to discuss a research paper, but she noticed a row of framed pictures that lined his window ledge. In one particular photograph, he and his wife were operating together. They were clad in full surgeon's attire—blue surgical gowns, caps, and face masks—their heads leaning in toward each other, their eyes fixed on the operative field below.

"I can tell it was quiet and serene," Stephanie said. "There was probably a slight beeping in the back. It's just the two of them working and it's just a calming photo. It's as though they are swans. The two swan heads that make a heart—that's what it reminds me of. They're working, but it's as if they're bonding."

When she met with her adviser to discuss her potential rank list, Stephanie mentioned the photo again. "I don't think that will be something I will be able to share with my spouse," she said, feeling disappointed. If she had been single, she later told me, perhaps she would have considered transplant surgery and put UCSF atop her list. But because she was in a serious relationship, children and a family seemed a reality to her—even if it would be seven to ten years until she could start one. So, with trembling voice and hands, she told her adviser she would rank Stanford, where a cancer surgeon she had known as an undergraduate would be a great mentor, at the top of her list, instead of UCSF.

By eliminating transplant from the possible surgical areas she would one day specialize in, all Stephanie had done was rule out arguably the single worst lifestyle in all of medicine. The rest of the surgery fields were not exactly family-friendly, either. Still, I felt guilt tighten my chest when she recounted the story.

"Do you feel like you're giving up something for me?" I asked.

"Well, a little bit," she said. "But it's worth it."

Stephanie hid around the corner as I placed the orchid in front of her adviser's open office door. It was an encounter she figured best to avoid that morning. Then Stephanie and I walked to the Golden Gate Room to pick up her envelope. If she landed her first or second choice—the latter I figured unlikely after the meeting with her adviser—we would have seven years in the Bay Area. Spot number three meant our life together would have to be in Boston. Number four and we would be moving to St. Louis. Five through eight and, well, I couldn't even remember. Not that it mattered. There was only one hospital listed in that envelope waiting for us and, in less than an hour, we would know.

At 8:30 A.M. on Match Day, the New York Medical College fourth-years in Manhattan boarded a charter bus bound for campus. Rakhi and Scott took seats near the back, just across the aisle from Michele and Ted. The four friends twisted their bodies to talk with each other and their classmates Tammy, Aaron, and

Ben, who made up the final row just behind them. Nerves translated into giddy chatter, filling the air and drowning out most of the lyrics to Jewel's "You Were Meant for Me" as it seeped from the bus's stereo system. Out the window, as they began to make their way north, a sign at Yankee Stadium counted down the twenty-six remaining days until a new season and a fresh start. Scott asked Rakhi how she was doing.

"You know when you're going on a roller coaster and you're going to the top, slowly, slowly, slowly, and you hear the *click, click, click, click* of the car going up, up, up to the top and then it falls? I kind of feel I'm slowly working my way up," Rakhi said. The gold earrings from India that she wore on special occasions dangled from her ears as she spoke. "I still feel like I'm halfway up. Not quite there yet."

"Before you're ready to plunge?" Scott asked.

"Yeah."

Across the aisle, sunglasses shielded Michele's eyes. She seemed in good spirits, teasing Ted when Aaron asked him how he was doing. "He doesn't have emotions," Michele said. Ted chuckled. He appeared the calmest of the group, turning to watch the others as they joked but remaining mostly quiet himself. Michele had asked him earlier how they should open their envelopes, and he had replied, wryly, "With our hands."

As the bus drew closer to campus, they passed the part of town where some of them had lived during their first year of medical school. They pointed to it, to each other, and shouted out memories. Then the bus entered campus. Red letters on a white banner blared from the side of the brick building: "New York Medical College Celebrates Senior Match Day." White tents stood on the lawn in front. They recognized the tents where they would flock after the ceremony's conclusion for beer, wine, and sandwiches. For years, they had crashed those Match Day parties.

The first time, Rakhi had not even known it was Match Day. She sat studying in the college's library, and lifted her head when she heard sudden shouts and cheers. The noise had struck her as out of place, a roar of a crowd that, to Rakhi's imagination, belonged more in a football stadium than a medical school. She had exchanged glances with two other first-year students and stood up to inspect the source of the commotion, leaving her notes and neuroscience textbook open on the table as she left the library. Only then had she discovered the envelopes, the tears, the celebrations, and the tents.

Now everyone on the bus seemed to digest that these tents were finally for them. Still, no one would see their interiors for several hours. While students in the West woke up and needed to wait only until 9 A.M., in the East there was plenty of time to let the imagination run before the noon ceremony. New York Medical College filled the morning with talks by students vying for the honor of graduation speaker. Sitting in the school's auditorium, they also voted on finalists for the Good Physician Award—to recognize the one classmate who best exemplified "those intangible qualities of the good physician." The finalists, to no surprise of her friends, would include Rakhi. She was gentle, sensitive, and cared deeply about every patient she saw. Rakhi had nominated and voted for her friend Sarah. But she felt touched to see her own name written among the finalists on a whiteboard that morning. It added to the overwhelming nature of the day. She and Scott remained in the auditorium after most of the other students left to mill about outside.

"I can't go out there yet," Rakhi said.

"Do you think the envelopes are out there yet?" Scott wondered out loud. The ceremony was still forty-five minutes away. "Are you feeling nervous?" he asked Rakhi.

"Yes, but excited at the same time," she said.

Outside, Michele and Ted stood with a cluster of friends. Across the lawn, one of their classmates sat at a picnic table by himself, his head down, hidden between his palms. "It sucks," Michele said. "I want to know now." She looked at the building. Some of the students had already migrated to the lobby, waiting. "Just standing in the middle there, you only have one thing to talk about."

Back when we were in college, I used to steal glimpses of Stephanie's hands. Her long, slender fingers were stunning and delicate. Even five years later, anytime we walked together I would reach for her hand, soft and smooth, and weave her fingers in between my own. Sometimes she would slide right out of my grasp, teasing me, waiting for my own hand to follow hers and hang on.

Stephanie's hands also were remarkably steady. I knew this from the times I had made her hold her arms straight out, hands next to mine. Someone had once told me that it was almost impossible to keep your hands completely still, and I decided to use a sample size of two to test this theory. My fingers fluttered ever so slightly. Stephanie's suspended still in the air. It was easy to imagine her hands gently tying surgical knots or wielding a scalpel with perfect precision. Even now, in the moments before she would learn her fate, her hands were perfectly still. They waited on the table. My sweaty palms and shaky fingers were their delegates.

Because everyone had already been instructed to retrieve their envelopes, there was little movement in UCSF's Golden Gate Room in those final seconds before Dean Kessler finally gave the green light. Then hands busied themselves with the task. Stephanie and I leaned in together. I removed a single folded white sheet of paper from the brown envelope. Our eyes cast downward on the black font. Under the big, bold headline 2006 MATCH RESULTS was the date. The next line listed her identification number. The next, her medical school code. The next, her name. I continued reading, past the program code, past the program name—general surgery—and down to the final line, labeled "institution name."

We were sitting. And then we were standing. Stephanie beamed. The room was suddenly alive again. People around us hugged, cried, screamed, and scurried between tables and chairs to find out how their friends had matched. Stephanie reached for her cell phone. I told her how proud I was of her. Then I asked her classmate to take our photograph. I wrapped my left arm around Stephanie. With my right, I pulled up my sweater to reveal the T-shirt underneath. Our photographer laughed. Stephanie turned around to see what I had done. I pointed to the shirt, proof that my confidence in her had been justified. Across its front, big red letters spelled STANFORD.

By 11:30 A.M., Michele, Ted, Rakhi, and Scott joined the crowded masses in New York Medical College's Medical Education Center. Nearly two hundred students crammed into the small lobby. A television news cameraman from the local ABC affiliate leaned over the staircase on the side. Pieces of paper taped to the walls dictated the stations where the students would eventually go to pick up their envelopes. A podium stood on one end for what the students assumed would be more speeches—this time from school administrators or professors—before the designated hour. Every few minutes, as more of the graduating students crowded into the lobby, the noise grew.

"Quiet down!" someone shouted. The dean walked to the podium and told the students what a good Match this year was for the school's students. Then she listed some of the results. "We had five appointments at Oregon and five at UCLA." She said, "There are four at Yale, and four at NYU. There are three each at UC–San Francisco—" Someone in the crowd gasped. The students had to be tallying the results in their heads. They painfully listened while the dean listed or, worse yet, omitted their first-choice hospitals and tried to remember who else in their class had wanted to go to the same place.

"I don't see a clock in here, but according to my watch, it's pretty close to 12:00 and so, if you'd like, you can go to—" The deans' final words were drowned out. Michele had been holding Ted's hand for much of the speech. Now she let it go to give Rakhi a brief hug. Then they parted for separate ends of the room. Waves of students flowed in every direction, trying to reach the edges where the school's staff held the thick piles of yellow and white envelopes.

Rakhi found the line forming in front of the sign labeled A–B. At the front, a woman handed her two envelopes. One would have a survey of some kind—it was mentioned during the speeches, when nobody could concentrate on the words spoken—and the other, the results. A scream erupted from the other end of the room. The roller-coaster ride had turned over the peak, students flinging their arms in the air. Shrieks rose from somewhere in the masses. Rakhi turned to Scott.

"Open this beige guy," he suggested.

She felt as if she was going to throw up. She tore at the envelope. Scott peered over her shoulder. "Oh. This is the survey," he said. "The other one, the other one!" Rakhi swapped envelopes, then ripped again. She pulled out a white piece of paper and unfolded it. Both her and Scott's eyes scanned the sheet, reading the first two letters—UC—and trying to translate the rest of the line.

Rakhi said it first, softly. Then she heard Scott shout the same—"UCLA!" She had been trying to convince herself all week that this is what she wanted. Now she turned to Scott and saw his eyes glistening. He reached out his arms and hugged her. All around, friends shouted the names of hospitals and universities—"CPMC!" and "Oregon? Oregon!" Rakhi looked out and smiled, cheering briefly for each one. Still, emotions came rushing out as her mascara mixed with tears. Her first choice had not wanted her. More cheers erupted. Students stood with cell phones attached to their ears and shouted into the mouthpieces. Others ran from classmate to classmate. One was upon Rakhi just seconds later.

"Where are you going to be?" he asked.

"UCLA."

"Congratulations, that's so awesome," he said in one breath, then turned to the next person. "You, buddy, what about you?"

Sounds bounced inside the lobby's walls. Screams continued to thunder from the steady roar of two hundred voices. It was impossible to digest anything. Scott said he was about to call Rakhi's parents to tell them the news, but Rakhi pleaded with him not to. Not yet. She needed to calm down. And she wanted to find out where Michele and Ted had matched.

Michele and Ted had needed to split up momentarily to retrieve their envelopes from different sides of the room. Michele had hers in hand first, then walked back to where she could see Ted picking up his own. Her hands shook as he returned to her. She opened first. She briefly read that she would spend her preliminary year in Danbury, Connecticut—that was fine—and scanned for where she matched for the four years of radiology. Westchester. Westchester! Her first choice! The words on her piece of paper blurred together as she started crying.

Then Ted opened his. All surrounding noise fell distant as his eyes darted across the page. *Okay, there's my name,* he thought. *And there's where the program is . . . Columbia.* It was Ted's second ranking, a practical tie for him with NYU when determining his rank list, and he smiled upon seeing the prestigious program. Michele hugged him, then gave him a kiss. The trip from Columbia to Westchester was nothing, Michele knew. Besides, she had figured she would live in Manhattan anyway and make the commute. Michele felt ecstatic. Ted told her that Rachlin was standing right behind her. Michele spun around.

"Are you happy?" Rachlin asked.

"Are you kidding?" Michele hugged her professor. She turned back to Ted to make sure he was not disappointed in landing his second choice. He assured her he wasn't. Then she thought to ask him about his preliminary year. Like Michele, as an anesthesiologist Ted would spend one preliminary year in medicine rotations before beginning rotations in his specialty.

Michele felt a tinge of disappointment as he told her he would be on Long Island. The hospital was an hour and a half from where she would live in Danbury for her first year. But she shrugged it off for now. Ted, too, felt relief. If he had landed his fourth choice instead of second, he would have had to buy a plane ticket to Los Angeles. And that would have meant a relationship talk with Michele. Now they could just enjoy this time. The two of them walked over to Rakhi and Scott. They shared results.

Michele hugged Rakhi and tried to comfort her. She whispered in Rakhi's ear. "This is how it was supposed to be," she said. "You did everything in your power. And you're going to be a great doctor."

Scott handed Rakhi the phone to talk to her parents. She listened for a moment, then—"I am, I am," she assured them. "I was a little sad right when I opened it. Just a little bit like, oh, I didn't get the first one, but this is the best thing for both of us. It really is. So it's the best in the end."

Riding on the bus back to Manhattan, Rakhi looked exhausted. Scott acknowledged her disappointment but also asked if she was excited. She told him yes. Mainly, she was excited to finally stop worrying. The chatter on the bus grew soft, and Rakhi stared out the window.

The nation had divvied up the latest class of doctors, as it had the year before, as it would do again in the same ritual one year later. Of the 15,008 graduating U.S. medical students who had submitted their rank lists in 2006, 14,059 received their marching orders that day. While Stephanie spoke with her mother, then my mother, then my grandparents, each wanting to congratulate her on landing her first choice, I called New York for an update from my friends. Overall, the computer algorithm seemed to make good on its promise, pairing everybody in our circle of friends with one of their top choices. Still, I knew the good of the whole did not ease individual disappointments or concerns.

That evening, Stephanie and I drove down the peninsula to Stanford through a trickling rain. We both knew the campus well from our undergraduate years, but with the new decree that the university would be our home for the next seven years, we felt the need to set foot on campus immediately to make it feel like a reality. About forty-five minutes after leaving San Francisco, we were in Palo Alto.

Stanford makes a strong first impression. Towering palm trees line a long and narrow road that serves as an entrance to campus. Red roofs dot the university's skyline, and sandstone buildings form a quadrangle in the center of the school's land. Everything about the campus seems proper and in its place. Perfectly mowed lawns stretch toward rows of red flowers, some clustered to form the letter S, and away from the palms, Campus Drive curves beneath the sprawling arms of oak trees. Bicycles cross every which way, past sand volleyball courts, fountains, Rodin sculptures, and up to the university's medical center.

We parked alongside the hospital. Stephanie walked with a sense of pride and ownership. This was her hospital. Here she would be Dr. Chao. Here she would care for patients; here she would work in the operating rooms. In the parking lot, she ran into an intern who recognized her from her student rotation at Stanford. He congratulated her on her match. He told her she was going to love it here. Around the corner, the red letters and white light of the emergency room sign cut through the dark night.

Surgical interns often entered the hospital before sunrise and left after sunset, and I wondered how much daylight Stephanie would see these next years. When we had looked in that envelope, I felt thrilled about moving back to California. I imagined bike rides together and hikes in the foothills. I thought of Stanford basketball games and barbeques with friends. We might have dinner at her parents' house one week and take a weekend drive to Los Angeles to visit my mother the next. It seemed perfect. But as we stood outside the hospital that night, I realized that I was still uncertain about the life of a resident. As this reality grew closer, all of my friends told me not to expect to see Stephanie very much. And when I did, they said, expect her to be exhausted.

5

Persian Rugs and Getting Pimped

Once, while Stephanie was on a residency interview, a surgeon told her an old saying that had been passed down for years. A good intern, he said, is like a Persian rug—meant to be walked all over and occasionally taken out back and beaten with a stick. Stephanie, Michele, and Rakhi were entering a new world with its own hierarchy (of which they would be at the bottom), its own rules, and even its own dangers. Older physicians were full of tales about residency. Among surgeons, the doctors who seemed to have the worst lifestyle as residents, I began to notice a common horror story.

When it happened to Fred Tibayan he was tired, but that was nothing unusual. Sleep was a luxury for residents. They closed their eyes when they could: while cooking something on the stove; for a moment in the bathroom; for a red light. Fred would sometimes shift his car into park while waiting at the traffic light so he could shut his eyes just for an instant, even though it meant prying them open seconds later. Other residents used the honks of horns as a green light's audible alarm.

Fred was an intelligent and even-tempered man with a sharp sense of humor. He frequently cited references from the classics he had read as an undergraduate at Harvard and from the graphic novels he continued to devour. Stephanie had met him during a month-long visiting rotation at Stanford while she was in medical school, and the two bonded despite their age difference. He had started his surgical residency a month or two after she had enjoyed her high school prom. Eight years later, when she finished medical school and matched at Stanford, he was completing his residency only to look forward to another three years of additional training in cardiothoracic surgery. In the eight years since starting residency, Fred had put on a few pounds and thanked God for TiVo, which kept him in touch with popular culture. He spent, he later guessed, somewhere between 110 and 120 hours at the hospital during most weeks of his intern year. Nobody counted. Most months, he was the on-call resident every third night— which meant, in addition to the day's work, staying at the hospital throughout the evening and into the next day. Working thirty-six hours on no sleep was not uncommon.

Stanford's residents rotated among four hospitals. All four had call rooms where, in the rare case of a quiet evening, residents on call overnight could retreat for catnaps in between dances with their pagers. The rooms were sparse, dusty, and often made up of a lonely twin bed, a lamp, and a bare desk. In one, a package of Maruchan instant ramen noodles and an alarm clock strangled by its own cord were hidden in a desk drawer. Fred spent plenty of nights as the overnight on-call resident in these rooms. By the bed in the VA he even taped up a photograph of Ol' Blue Eyes,

Frank Sinatra, to add a little warmth. But whenever he chose to sleep in the hospital when he could have gone home, even for a fraction of the night, he felt robbed. His pasty mouth reminded him that he had not brushed his teeth. One step out of bed and it was right back to work. Days blurred together, distinguished only by the changing numbers on the hospital orders that a resident dated. So, like most residents, no matter how tired he was, if Fred was not designated as the in-house call resident, he made an effort to drive home to sleep. Even if just for a few hours.

On the day it happened to Fred, he had just finished at the Santa Clara Valley Medical Center. He lived in campus housing, just blocks from the university's main hospital. But during rotations at either of the two hospitals in Santa Clara, long shifts ended with at least a half-hour drive home, assuming traffic was forgiving. On this day, Fred exited the Interstate 280 and made his way down the narrow roads on Stanford's edge. The road curved around the university's pristine golf course. Just five minutes from his apartment, his eyes grew heavy. Darkness. Then, a Nissan Maxima. Fred slammed on the brakes and turned the wheel hard. He hit the back of the Nissan. His air bag exploded. His vehicle stopped in a ditch by the side of the road.

It was as if someone had injected him with Adrenalin. Fred went from complete exhaustion to feeling wired. He jumped out of his car and made sure he had not hurt anyone, then considered himself lucky. He wiped away blood from the cuts on his hands and head, caused by the broken glass. Moments later, a Stanford doctor drove by and leaned out of the car to see if Fred was okay. Fred waved him off. He told him he was fine. The last thing Fred wanted was to be brought into his own hospital as a trauma patient.

As Stephanie prepared for residency, I often worried that she would fall asleep driving home from a night on call. I pleaded with her that, if she ever felt too tired to drive, she should call me. I would pick her up. It was not just the anecdotes from our friends that worried me. The risk of an overtired intern seemed to be a popular topic in academic journals. One article equated hand-eye coordination impairment after being awake for twenty-four hours to that caused by a blood alcohol level of .10 percent, above the legal driving limit. Another claimed that self-reported rates of car crashes among residents were three times that of nonresident drivers. And in a letter to the editor of *The Journal of the American Medical Association,* two doctors from Irvine, California, noted that, of the seven surgical residents they interviewed in their hospital, six had fallen asleep driving to or from work during internship year and three had been in accidents.

In some residency programs, it was easy for an intern to live in or near the hospital. Michele would move into a hospital-owned apartment at the edge of Danbury Hospital's parking lot for the year. But when a program's residents rotated at multiple hospitals, it complicated the issue of where to find housing. In Los Angeles, Rakhi and Scott were also moving into campus housing, just a short drive from UCLA's main hospital. But at least one rotation would require Rakhi to drive the city's congested freeways for a longer distance. At Stanford, I was less worried about Stephanie's ten-minute commute up University Avenue to the university's hospital than I was about the odds of her getting safely to and from the Santa Clara hospitals.

This danger, of course, stemmed from the long hours a resident worked. In addition to the constant exhaustion, a resident's work hours eliminated most other facets of life. At many hospitals, it seemed that residents were not expected to have much of a life away from work. Articles in medical journals detailed tales of depression and failed marriages. Of course, medical students knew this getting into the field. For the years of residency, their lives would not be their own.

There were a variety of opinions on why residents needed to work so many hours. Some viewed it as tradition and a test of survival, ensuring that only the strongest practiced medicine. It no doubt discouraged some people from applying to the more demanding fields. Others speculated that residents were exploited because they were cheap labor. Medicare gave money to teaching hospitals to help pay for residents and graduate medical education. By 2006, a first-year resident's salary at most hospitals averaged just over $43,000, enough to cover rent and groceries. But given the number of hours they worked, their salary was low enough to lead a CBS MarketWatch columnist in 2003 to list residents among the ten most underpaid jobs in the country. Most residents did not want to depress themselves by thinking about their salaries in terms of hourly rates, especially with the hundreds of thousands of dollars they still owed in college and medical school loans. But the columnist did, noting that their hourly wage was roughly the equivalent of that of a restaurant dishwasher. There was no overtime pay. And while residents did get some vacation, they were not entitled to national holidays or full weekends. So, in one regard, a hospital was getting a bargain. A nurse practitioner or another physician doing the same work would prove more costly.

But this was a cynic's view. Two other explanations were more common: the long hours were necessary to give residents enough experience and exposure to a wide variety of cases, and the extended hours led to the best quality of care for a patient. The long hours enabled residents to continue to care for patients they had admitted much earlier in the day and to monitor the course of the disease as a result of the treatments they themselves rendered, rather than simply hand off the responsibility to the next resident.

To a new intern about to start in 2006—or to their significant other and family members, for that matter—twenty-four-hour shifts and eighty-hour workweeks still sounded pretty daunting. To the older generation, though, it seemed as if the newcomers were getting off easy. That's because a drastic change had taken place throughout the nation's residency programs in 2003, just three years before Stephanie, Michele, and Rakhi joined the working world of doctors. It began with a tragedy in New York that grabbed the nation's attention. This led to one giant question: if residents were so sleep deprived, what did that mean for the lives they cared for?

Late one Sunday evening in March 1984, Sidney Zion and his wife brought their daughter Libby to the emergency room at New York Hospital. The eighteen-year-old had a fever and had looked ill enough for her brother to call his parents home from a party. By the time Libby arrived at the hospital, her fever was 103 degrees. She had been shaking for much of the car ride and continued to do so at the hospital, her head, arms, and legs sporadically jerking.

The past few days had been difficult for Libby, between a dentist's removal of her infected tooth and the development of an earache, in addition to the fever. In the emergency room, when the doctors took her medical history and asked what medication she was on, Libby and her mother told them of an antibiotic she had been prescribed, as well as the antidepressant she regularly took. The doctors also noted that she had a high white blood cell count, which hinted at an infection. They performed tests to try to figure out what was causing the fever but came up with no clear answers.

Sidney grew frustrated. He was a well-connected journalist in New York and a former attorney who considered Frank Sinatra a friend. He had written for *The New York Times* and *The New York Post*. Earlier in the evening, when he first came home and saw his daughter, he had called a physician he knew at the doctor's home. Dr. Raymond Sherman, an attending at New York Hospital, advised Sidney to bring Libby to the hospital's emergency room. At the hospital, the doctor who examined Libby consulted with Dr. Sherman over the phone, and they decided the hospital should admit Libby. But Sidney would later note that none of the "pros" had been there. The doctors who Libby saw were residents.

Libby was moved to the fifth floor, and her care was transferred to the residents on call—an intern named Luise Weinstein and a second-year resident, Gregg Stone. As an intern, Dr. Weinstein was less than a year out of medical school, and her workweek averaged between 95 and 110 hours. That evening, she was responsible for about forty patients and had been on duty for close to eighteen hours by the time Libby was brought upstairs. Sometime near 3 A.M., with Libby's condition appearing to remain the same and the doctors keeping her under observation, Sidney and his wife, Elsa, went home. The next morning, they got a phone call from the hospital. Libby had died.

Though reports vary, it seemed that, in the ensuing hours,

Libby had tried to climb out of bed and continued to jerk. Dr. Weinstein prescribed the painkiller Demerol to treat her agitation and shivering, and later ordered restraints and an injection of a tranquilizer. For several hours, Dr. Weinstein was busy tending to other patients and, when called by the nurse regarding Libby's condition, had given orders over the phone. By 6:30 A.M., Libby's fever was more than 106 degrees. Ten minutes later, she went into cardiac arrest. Nurses and doctors spent almost an hour trying to revive her.

What caused Libby's death is a subject that has been debated for years. In recounting it in his book *When Illness Goes Public,* Dr. Barron H. Lerner, a professor of medicine and public health at Columbia University, noted that as many as five stories were told over the years to explain the death. Some from the hospital first claimed the death was not preventable, and later speculated that Libby might have concealed cocaine use. Sidney believed they were trying to blame the victim and that errors and neglect had killed his daughter. An unsupervised, overworked intern and second-year resident had made mistakes, he claimed. His grief manifested in anger. By publicly pointing the finger at the hospital, he also brought the ways of medical residency—the long hours and inexperienced doctors making crucial life-or-death decisions—to the public's attention. He mounted an aggressive campaign. He filed a malpractice suit against multiple doctors and the hospital. He also convinced Manhattan's district attorney to convene a grand jury for possible criminal indictments. While the grand jury did not hand down any indictments, it issued a report that was, as later described by two doctors in *The New England Journal of Medicine,* "an indictment of American graduate Medical Education."

The grand jury report criticized the hospital for not moving the patient to the intensive care unit and for prescribing Demerol, a drug that might cause complications when mixed with the antidepressant. But the report suggested that the conditions leading to Libby Zion's death existed at other hospitals as well. Among others, the jury's report included recommendations regarding supervision of residents and work hours. As a result, New York's state health commissioner and governor put together a committee of nine physicians to study the grand jury's suggestions and recommend changes to the state's hospitals and residency programs.

Meanwhile, two discussions ensued. The public, outraged that the doctors caring for them were so sleep deprived, seemed to fixate on the work hours. The medical community, set in its ways, split on the issue of whether long hours led to costly errors such as Libby Zion's death. "The grand jury's recommendations were motivated by a desire to improve hospital care," Drs. David Asch and Ruth Parker wrote in *The New England Journal of Medicine* in 1988. "But the grand jury confused professional incompetence with long working hours."

After eighteen months, the committee of doctors that came to be known as the Bell Commission—after its chair, Dr. Bertrand Bell—made its recommendations. Most involved the issue of supervision, but it was the recommendation that residents be restricted to an average of no more than eighty hours in a workweek—a number Bell and a colleague came up with while sitting on his porch one day—that got the most attention. In 1989 New York changed its health code. Among other rules, it became the first state to limit residents to eighty-hour workweeks.

By the mid-1990s, Sidney Zion's malpractice suit against the hospital played out in front of the nation on Court TV, only increasing the attention to the practices of medical education. The public's concern grew. An inspection of New York hospitals found that they frequently violated the new regulations. More stories on resident work hours appeared in the media as the century turned: *Time* magazine ran a piece, and the CBS news program *60 Minutes* rebroadcast its examination of the issue from 1987. The Health Research Group, the same advocacy group that had called for a change to the Match's algorithm, now in coordination with the Committee of Interns and Residents and the American Medical Student Association, filed a petition with the U.S. Department of Labor in 2001. In it, they asked that the Occupational Safety and Health Administration implement similar regulations on work hours for the entire nation's residents as New York had done, noting the intent of "providing more humane and safe working conditions for medical residents and fellows, which will result in a better standard of care for all patients." And Representative John Conyers Jr., a congressman from Michigan, worked on a bill that would put the authority to regulate resident work hours in the government's hands.

By 2002, the Accreditation Council for Graduate Medical Education, responsible for the accreditation of the nation's residency programs, got involved. With the public convinced that the longer hours compromised patient safety, and with the threat of a possible government regulation, the council set limits on hours for residency programs across the country. A resident's workweek could not exceed eighty hours, when averaged over four weeks. They were not to work more than twenty-four straight hours, though they were given an additional six hours of waffle room for "continuity of care and education" purposes. They were to have ten hours off in between shifts. And they were to have one day free in seven, also averaged over four weeks. The rules went into place in July 2003.

It was hard for me to imagine many professions questioning whether an eighty-hour week was enough. And it was also hard to believe that, with lives at stake, a hospital would want anything other than well-rested doctors. But by the time Stephanie, Michele, and Rakhi began residency, the debate over the new work hours, already in place, was three years strong. Surprisingly, conclusions were mixed as to the effect of the new rules on over-all patient mortality, with conflicting or insufficient data. Both sides could point to studies they felt proved their point. Academic journal articles concluded, as they often did, by calling for more research.

In June 2006, Stanford held an orientation for its new surgical residents, Stephanie among them. There, administrators handed the wide-eyed recent graduates piles of papers. One instructed them on how to report their hours. The way in which hospitals collected a resident's hours was not uniform across the country, and a *Journal of the American Medical Association* study showed that 83 percent of the interns surveyed in the year after the rules changed had reported work hours that did not meet the new standards during at least one month. But Stephanie's residency program made a point to note the importance of the work-hour rules at the orientation. If residents were late in reporting their hours, they would be locked out of the computer system and have to see a department administrator about getting back in. Stephanie was to log on to a Web site regularly and report when she had gone in and when she had gone out of the hospital each day.

Medicine, some elder statesmen complained, should not be shift work. Even Fred, who benefited from the new rules during his last three years of residency, believed that the clock-in, clock-out mentality led residents to feel less ownership over a given patient's care. He admitted that the new rule of an average of one day off per week was a good thing. It made it easier for the interns to deal with life outside the hospital. There had been times during his residency when Fred had not paid his bills on time. His lights and phone had been turned off. During his own internship year he could go four or five months without a full day off, and when he did get one, or even on occasion two, it was a precious gift he would never forget. Two weekend days off in a row was a rarity so treasured, residents called it a "golden weekend." But Fred questioned the other rules, particularly the one that sent a resident home after thirty hours. "Some people think they will turn into a pumpkin after thirty hours and have to go home or they will start killing patients," he once reflected. "This is not true."

The debate over work hours divided the generations. To the old, the young seemed more concerned about lifestyle than hard work. There was no place for worrying about clocking out at a certain hour. Endurance through long weeks with limited time off was the way it had always been done. Older doctors went through the hellish training, and they expected the next generation to be equally dedicated, equally single-minded. To the young, the old looked set in their ways and probably proud of having walked to school uphill, both ways, in the snow. At risk, some argued, was patient safety.

To cut the residents' workweeks from as many as one-hundred-plus hours for some to eighty, as well as address the issue that no resident could work more than thirty hours straight, many hospitals came to rely on what is called cross coverage and instituted a night float system. For a designated period of time, from a week to a month, a resident would be assigned to night float. He or she typically arrived at the hospital at five or six in the evening and received signout—updates on each patient on the service—from the daytime interns. A surgery program, for example, might have two of its night float surgery interns each cover four of the departments' services, such as trauma or transplant, whereas during the daytime, each service would have its own intern. By about six or seven in the morning, the night float intern would give signout back to each of the returning daytime interns, telling them of any changes that occurred overnight. On other days, or on rotations without a night float, interns could still take overnight call, staying twenty-four hours from one morning until the next.

On other rotations, a hospital might institute home call for interns and residents. In these cases, the young doctors left their pagers turned on for multiple nights each week while they were at home. When the pager did not sound, they were not working. When it beeped, they called the hospital and tried to handle patient care over the phone with verbal orders to the nurses. These often entailed simple orders like supplemental pain medicine or stool softeners and laxatives. But if the call required more attention, they routinely drove back to the hospital and only then logged the hours toward the eighty-hour limit.

Teaching hospitals referred to interns and residents as house officers. The interns were the first line of care for most patients, and good interns knew their patients better than anybody else.

They knew what time they last urinated, when they had their last bowel movement, and when they last passed gas—all important signs that the body was working properly. They "pre-rounded" on patients in the early morning, visiting each one in advance of the morning rounds they would do with the rest of the medical team. They looked over charts and vital signs and made sure the nurses had filled all orders for medications. Then they presented the patients to their more senior residents on rounds. Often these times were used for teaching purposes as well as patient care. The attending physicians "pimped" the residents, a form of the Socratic method, grilling them with questions about the patient's disease process, etiology of the disease, or even medical minutiae while standing outside the patient's room or at the foot of the bed. After rounds, the interns noted what their senior doctors had dictated. They wrote orders into charts or entered them into a computer system and called consultants from other medical services accordingly. If they had time during the day, they might circle the ward from one patient's room to the next, to be the first to discover any subtle changes in their patients' conditions.

Their pagers constantly sounded throughout the day, interrupting work with more work. Senior residents paged them when there were new patients to see. Nurses paged them when the status on any of their patients changed and required action. The interns sometimes needed to make on-the-spot decisions, or call a more senior resident if they had questions. "And remember," some doctors were known to joke, "asking for help is a sign of weakness."

But more than anything, the interns' days were about their lists. Every intern carried one. They folded a piece of paper that had the names and room numbers of their patients and the bare essentials of each case printed on the front. On it, they scribbled their To-Dos. Helping their patients was the ultimate goal. Still, it was difficult to remain compassionate as their list of patients grew. Each additional patient meant more pre-rounding in the morning, later evenings at the hospital, and less sleep. With new patients constantly arriving, residents looked to discharge those who were able to go home. If a patient grew worse, they might hope their senior residents would "turf" the patient to another service. Discharging patients was inevitably on their minds. Some interns called discharging all of the patients on their list "winning the game." On top of these duties, surgical interns tried to get valuable time in the operating rooms to learn from their attending doctors and assist with cases.

In the early months, the juggling act would take longer. Stephanie's first day would be a Wednesday, and because she suspected the week would be averaged into the four-week period as if it had been a full week, she was not worried about her hours. She would begin at Stanford Hospital at 4:30 in the morning on what just so happened to be the summer solstice—the longest day of the year. She said she was excited to begin, but she also sounded tense. When I could not understand something she said that night, I asked her again. "I don't have time to repeat things twice," she told me, frenzied. She needed to get to bed. She set her alarm for 3:50 A.M. Eventually, she figured, she would get faster at pre-rounding on patients. Then she might be able to go in at 5:00 A.M.

"Nothing like having to pre-round at 4 A.M. to make you more efficient," Fred liked to say.

In medical school, clinical rotations allowed third-year and fourth-year students to feel what it was like to work in a hospital. But medical students could always look to the residents to guide them, to co-sign any hospital orders for them, and to double-check their work. As their own residencies began, that feeling of security would vanish. When they walked into rooms, patients would look up from the beds and see doctors.

Early in the morning, on Wednesday, June 21, 2006, Stephanie's cell phone made three short beeps. She looked down and saw she had a text message. It was from Fred. "Welcome to your first day," it said. "Try not to kill anyone."

6

Becoming Doctor

Palo Alto's University Avenue did not quite awaken at four in the morning as much as it opened its groggy eyes, rolled over, and drifted off again. A row of traffic lights flashed the yellow of a machine on sleep mode. Storefronts for Michael's Gelato and Siam Royal, for University Café and Mills the Florist slumbered in darkness. Empty parking spots left the normally crowded road looking bare and abandoned. Street-cleaning trucks broke a thick silence with whirls and swishes, then faded away, the only indication of their existence the quickly drying streaks on black asphalt. At its very end, where the avenue no longer needed its name to advertise the destination, street signs changed to Palm Drive and the road stretched inside Stanford's campus. There, the moon still hung above the Memorial Church mosaic.

Stephanie pulled her Volkswagen into the fourth aisle of the parking lot across the street from the hospital's emergency room entrance. It proved helpful, she quickly learned, to park in the same location every day so that fourteen hours later, when she finally walked outside again, she could turn off her brain rather than stand dumbstruck, having forgotten where she had left her car. She chose the fourth aisle in particular because it was closest to the walkway that crossed the street and continued on to the hospital. Her new life was about efficiency. Every minute saved meant a minute gained for sleeping, and it only took Stephanie a few days to memorize the timing of her daily trip. Seven minutes to drive from her apartment to the parking lot. Three minutes to walk from the parking lot to the hospital's entrance. One minute and thirty seconds to stride from the entrance to the D2 hallway, where the residents shared a small workroom complete with a stained and musty denim couch, two telephones, and three computers.

She walked briskly, a pace she would keep the entire day. On her feet, she wore dark maroon clogs. The shoes had felt comfortable during long hours of standing in medical school and could easily hide bloodstains. As she entered the hospital as a doctor for the first time, she dressed the part. She wore blue scrubs and her new white coat. On its left side, just below the lapel, red embroidered letters spelled STANFORD HOSPITAL in cursive. Stephanie had scored one of the white coats at the hospital with a belt attached to its back. She liked that it created something of a waistline, though as she walked, the pockets sagged from their contents—trauma shears, gauze, paper tape, alcohol pads, a scut list of patient-related To-Dos, a Pharmacopoeia guide, a cheat sheet she had printed on a three-by-five index card reminding her of normal lab values, and a pack of sutures to practice tying surgical knots should any free time arise. She also shoved her stethoscope in the coat's pocket. That was one way you could distinguish a surgeon from another doctor.

Internal medicine residents typically draped the stethoscopes over their necks. Some anesthesiologists hung it from a holster on the hip. Surgeons, Stephanie was told in medical school, kept the stethoscope in the coat pocket.

Excitement and anxiety mixed in Stephanie's stomach. She did not think of heroics or saving lives; she simply wanted to be safe. Before falling asleep the night before, she prayed that she would not hurt any patients. Now, on her first day of residency, Stephanie entered the workroom and paged the night float. Months later, she would learn to further maximize her time by talking to the night float resident on her cell phone during the drive to the hospital, teaching herself to remember anything important and write it down after she parked. But on this day, she sat at a desk, took out the patient list, and paged him. The resident called a moment later. "Welcome," he told her. Then, "So here's what happened to your patients last night."

The very existence of residency seemed proof that medical school did not fully prepare people to become doctors. Medical school graduates needed experience and guidance. And yet there was no easing into this job. Interns were immediately assigned and expected to care for patients. They needed to behave like doctors on day one and convince patients and staff of their competence, even if it was impossible to predict when these wide-eyed rookies would actually transform from civilians into competent physicians.

Stephanie and the other interns debated how they were supposed to respond to their pagers. They knew to call the phone number immediately, but they disagreed on what was the proper way to introduce themselves on the phone. Some wanted to be addressed by their new title. Stephanie thought about dialing and announcing, "Hello, this is Dr. Chao," but it sounded wrong. She did not know enough to be a doctor. Plus, plenty of the nurses who would page her were older and more experienced. It just felt more appropriate to introduce herself as Stephanie.

Her first month's rotation was made up mostly of surgical on-cology patients. Rounds with the more senior doctors began every morning at six so that they would finish in time to get to the oper-ating rooms for the day's surgeries, which typically began an hour or hour and a half later. They gathered just outside the first pa-tient's door or formed a semicircle of white coats at the foot of a bed. The intern needed to present each patient's case succinctly to the chief resident, as the most senior residents were called. On this rotation the chief was a former marine whose frequent rally-ing cry was "Get 'er done." He was efficient and competent and expected the same from the intern on the service, even on the first day. To prepare, the intern needed to visit every patient be-fore rounds began to check on their status and note any impor-tant changes. And because rounds began at six, and because the marine considered 6:01 late, Stephanie knew to be ready, notes in hand, at 5:59 A.M. That meant pre-rounding on her own at 4:30 A.M.

The escalators stood still at that early hour. The hallway lights remained dim. Despite the appearance of tranquillity, the hos-pital's halls were almost never quiet. A cacophony of dings and beeps flooded from heart monitors at the nurses' stations and from pulse oximeters through the open doors of patient rooms. If the monitors detected something wrong, their beeps increased in speed. Every now and then what sounded like a soda can slam-ming to the bottom of a vending machine indicated that nurses had sent paperwork, labs, or medications through the hospital's vacuum system. The nurses sat at desks in the middle of the halls and, on occasion, a police officer guarded a criminal's room just down the way.

Even if patients could sleep through the beeps, bangs, and dings, the hospital was not a place for getting rest. Doctors and nurses frequently entered the room to ask questions, to poke, prod, and inspect. And at four or five in the morning, Stephanie was no exception, waking up any patients still sleeping.

She had already looked up the vital signs for each patient after getting off the phone with the night float resident. The computers generated a short list of the past twenty-four hours' worth of vitals for all patients, but only after six A.M., so in order to pre-round earlier, Stephanie had checked each vital one by one: she read her patients' temperatures, blood pressure, pulse, and respiratory rates. She inspected how much fluid they took in and how much fluid they put out. She talked with their nurses to see how the patients did overnight. But she dreaded the last step of pre-rounds: waking up patients recovering from surgery. Many looked small and fragile beneath their blankets. Some mustered the strength for a cheery, "Good morning, Doctor," after opening their eyes. Stephanie checked the incisions to see how they were healing. She inquired if the patients were able to pass gas, a way to learn if their digestive systems were working. She asked them about their pain. Sometimes, as she spoke, she reached out and gently placed her hand on their arm or on the covers over their legs. Then she moved on to the next room. She was able to spend about five minutes with each person.

It felt as if she was always moving. There was no time to eat. Some interns carried nutrition bars in their white coats. Others scavenged for food at the nursing stations. A few even snacked on the leftovers of food trays abandoned by patients. Stephanie tried to bring food from home, but rarely got around to eating it. Months later, on her pediatric surgery rotation, she would resort to eating the Nature's Goodness baby food stocked in the pediatric floor pantry. She often grew dehydrated from not drinking enough. The benefit, though unintended, was she did not have to stop to use the bathroom. She briskly walked from room to room and often played with a needle driver in her pocket, practicing how to open and close the scissorslike surgeon's tool used for stitching up a wound.

As she finished rounds with the team on her first day, Stephanie went to the nurse's station. She wanted to sit for a moment to enter orders into the computer and update patient charts with progress notes. The notes, kept in thick binders on a cart by the nurses' station, detailed all doctors' examinations of patients and the plans for treatment and care. That way, anyone who needed information on a patient could easily look it up. A few minutes into writing these notes and orders, though, her pager beeped. Stephanie reached for the nearest phone and dialed the number.

"Hello, this is Stephanie," she said when a voice answered. It was her chief resident. He told her to get to the operating room. A lymph node biopsy would start in a few minutes, and she needed to assist. Stephanie raced to the operating room on the hospital's second floor. She knew from medical school that a resident should meet the patient in the pre-op area and answer any last minute questions, then possibly even wheel the patient into the operating room. But by the time she got there, both the patient and attending physician were already in the O.R. Stephanie was late.

Before she could begin, she needed to scrub in. She had learned the ritual dance in medical school, intended to rid her hands and forearms of bacteria. The operating room's scrub nurse made sure every instrument and person working on the patient remained sterile to decrease the chance of patient infection. A metal trough sat just outside the room. Stephanie leaned into the knee pedal to turn on the water. She took the presoaped sponge and washed, then tore at her arms, hands, and under her nails with the bristles on the flip side. With her elbows bent at ninety degrees and her hands in the air, water dripped down her forearms. She walked into the operating room. A nurse handed her a sterile blue towel, helped her put on the sterile gown, then tied it in the back.

The operating room looked much like the ones she had seen in medical school: sterile instruments sat on cloth-covered tables; bright light fixtures hung from the ceiling and illuminated the table beneath. Surgeons stood under the beams for hours, dressed in sterile gowns over their scrubs. The gowns and lights were a big part of why operating rooms were always kept so cold. If the room were any warmer, sweat would drip beneath the surgeons' face masks. And, as some overtired residents liked to joke, the cold air kept them awake. Blue towels draped over the patient, covering all but a square area where the surgeons would operate.

The attending doctor told Stephanie to make the incision. As a medical student, she had never made the first cut. During her times in an operating room, she had been mostly relegated to suction and retracting tools. It was nice that this doctor automatically assumed she could do it, but Stephanie held the scalpel with some uncertainty. Her life as a working doctor was no more than three and a half hours old.

"You're holding the scalpel wrong," the attending told her. "Hold it like a pencil."

Stephanie had the handle of the blade tucked in the palm of her hand, her fingers wrapping over the instrument. That was how she had been taught to hold a scalpel in medical school. She felt nervous. "I don't know exactly what you mean by that," she said.

The doctor took the scalpel out of Stephanie's hands and proceeded to do the incision herself.

The first months of internship are about uncertainty and fear. The operating room could be rough at times—a surgeon once barked at Stephanie, "Hold it like you're a surgeon!"—but at least there was always an attending doctor there, guiding the intern. Working nights on the patient floors, on the other hand, an intern could feel alone.

Periodically, Stephanie got paged during her night float shifts about patients recently out of surgery who experienced chest pain or whose oxygen saturations were dropping. These were the patients that made Stephanie start to sweat. Because she had not cared for these people during the daytime, it was harder to recognize patterns, to know what was normal for them or what was an indication of a larger problem. From a snapshot in time—a call from the nurse, a quick visit to the patient—she had to decide the severity of a medical issue. Just a few months out of medical school, with little experience, that was not an easy thing to do.

Eighty percent of her work at the hospital, she guessed, was checking up on patients, writing orders for fluids or safety restraints, and scribbling prescriptions. Vicodin, Colace, morphine, and Ativan were regulars. These were the calls she was more comfortable taking. Still, you could take nothing for granted. Rumors spread of how one hospital's intern once prescribed so much Ativan, a drug used for sedation, the nurses had to call "Code Blue" over the public address system to summon an emergency response team. As a medical student on rotations, Stephanie had needed her prescriptions and orders to be co-signed by a resident. Now, she saw, there was rarely someone watching over her shoulder. "I'm not that much smarter than I was as a student," she told me one day after work. "Yesterday I had a resident. Today it's me."

The first time Stephanie began a night float shift, another resident gave her a list of things to keep in mind. Number one: "You can't win." Number two: "Don't try to be a hero." Other items on the list reminded her that bladder scanners were always available, that transfers fresh out of the intensive care unit could easily code, and suggested that she learn how to read EKGs. It was not all glamour—number three on the list reminded her to get the breakfast cart at 6 A.M. for the other doctors. Stephanie took a red pen and circled the seventh item. "Don't hesitate to call your chief—but depending on your chief they won't like it."

Early one morning, at about 2 A.M., while Stephanie worked as the night float, a nurse paged her. A patient was complaining of chest pain. Stephanie went off to see him. The patient was about seventy years old. When Stephanie asked him about the chest pain, he mentioned that this was the first time he had ever felt it, a crushing sensation that made it hard for him to breathe. She decided to do a workup for a heart attack. She ordered an EKG. She gave him morphine, oxygen, aspirin, and ordered nitroglycerin. Students were often taught to remember these steps with the mnemonic M.O.A.N. Others learned it as M.O.N.A.B. with the reminder to include beta-blockers. Stephanie started the patient on beta-blockers to control his heart rate and reduce the stress on the heart, and she ordered labs. Then she knew not to be too confident in her response. For something this serious, she decided to let the surgical fellow know now, despite the hour.

Stephanie went to the cart and pulled out the patient's chart. The intern who had signed out at the end of the day had not mentioned who to call if something happened. There was no chief on this service, but there were two surgical fellows—the physicians just above chief residents in a hospital's hierarchy—and one of them had operated on the man just that evening. She decided he would be the most informed doctor regarding this patient, and paged him.

When her phone rang, Stephanie heard a sleepy voice on the other end. She told the fellow about the patient's chest pain and how she had responded.

"Okay," he said. "Did you already try calling the third-year resident?' he asked. Stephanie could tell he was not happy.

"No," she said.

"Did you try calling the other fellow?"

"No," she said. "I called you first because I didn't know who to call and I thought you had just operated on him."

"It will serve you well in your career in the future to go up the chain of command and to know who to call at night," he said.

Stephanie apologized. As an intern, she knew she would never win battles so there was no point in picking them. You just apologized. She asked him if he wanted her to call the other fellow and he said no, not now that she had already woken him up. She asked him if she should call the cardiology team to consult with and he said yes.

"Anything else you'd like me to do?" Stephanie asked.

"No" came the reply. Stephanie hung up. She knew she was right to have called, but still felt like an idiot. A few minutes later, when she woke the cardiologist to tell him about the patient, he thanked her for the call. He told her she had done everything right.

On the other side of the country, Michele also donned the new white coat and the role that came with it. She stood in the emergency room at Connecticut's Danbury Hospital and waited for the voice from above. It was the instant during which most of the hospital's doctors held their breath. They had heard a click from an overhead speaker and knew the public-address system had been activated. A moment later, an operator might utter one of a variety of messages to the hospital's staff. If it was late in the day, the voice instructed listeners that visiting hours were now over. If a patient had a medical emergency, the operator called for Code 99. On this day, the operator alerted the physicians to a Code Green.

There is only some uniformity to the code systems used by the nation's hospitals. Code Blue is most common for a medical emergency or cardiac arrest, but understanding one hospital's codes after training at another institution is like learning to think in a foreign language. An abducted child might prompt an overhead call of Code Pink in some places and Code Lindbergh in others. Code White might imply a bomb threat at one hospital or a pediatric emergency at another. Upon their arrival, new residents and staff usually received a small index card listing colors and the corresponding emergencies. At Danbury, Michele believed, Code Green, like Code 99, was a medical emergency, but in the E.R. rather than the patient's room.

The paramedics rushed a middle-aged man into the room. He had collapsed in the hospital parking lot. He lay unresponsive on the gurney. An emergency room attending doctor rushed to his side as they lifted the patient onto a bed. A whirlwind of activity followed anytime a code was called. Scrubs and white coats charged down hallways and came from all directions. Michele's attending physician "ran the code," commanding the fast-moving medical professionals and trying to bring some order to the chaos. He barked instructions, called for medications, and checked the chest monitors. Michele stood in the corner, not sure of her role. Even though Match Day had proved her successful in the quest to become a radiologist, her preliminary year was made up of almost no radiology work. Instead, she was scheduled to spend the first year rotating through other departments, with much of the year dominated by internal medicine work. Her career as a doctor began with the two-week rotation in emergency medicine.

Four or five nurses swirled around the patient. One drew blood. One dug through the patient's personal items to figure out his name. A respiratory therapist squeezed a flexible pumplike air bag hooked up to a mask to send air in and out of his lungs. And two nurses traded off pounding on the man's chest. Michele stood to the side. Nobody called for her help. Nobody instructed her on what to do.

Medical students rarely got close enough to see how codes worked, with so many people standing between them and the patient. But Michele was a doctor now, and she took the initiative.

She removed her white coat to free up her arms, and put on a set of gloves. Then she walked over to the nurse giving the patient chest compressions and offered to relieve her. Tired from the physical strain, the nurse agreed.

The bed was raised high and Michele stretched on the tip of her toes to reach the patient's chest. She put her right hand over the top of her left and interlaced her fingers. She straightened her arms and locked her elbows. Then she pushed her hands onto the man's chest, directly between his nipples. She pushed them again. Then again. She thought back to her instruction from medical school. She had to use enough force to press his chest down two inches, hard enough that ribs sometimes cracked. And she needed to make one hundred compressions in a minute, more than one every second. The pattern medical school had taught her was thirty compressions between every two breaths. Michele started counting the compressions. One. Two. Three. Four. But as she pounded on the unconscious patient, she watched the respiratory therapist squeeze the oxygen bag more frequently than she had expected, what seemed like every three or four seconds. She could not figure how she was to get thirty compressions before the therapist's next squeeze. This was not the protocol, she thought.

It became clear to Michele that, in real life, emergency responses might not always feel scripted. Residency would take adapting and learning on the fly. She stopped counting. She focused only on leaning into the man's chest, hard and fast.

Even if an intern knew what to do, part of the transformation from recent medical graduate to doctor seemed to be about exuding confidence. Without experience, that was hard for an intern to do. Yet for a new female doctor, there was an extra hurdle. Walking into patients' rooms, Stephanie realized, she was usually mistaken for a nurse. This did not especially irk her, nor did she mind how some of the older male patients called her sweetie or commented on her looks. But there were times when she felt an extra burden to overcome to reach that confidence, a burden she doubted her male peers felt.

One weekend in July, while Stephanie was the on-call intern in the hospital overnight, a nurse paged her at 3 A.M. One of Stephanie's patients was acting up, the nurse said. He was an eighty-year-old man who had been admitted to the hospital for a carotid endarterectomy—a surgery to remove deposits of fat from the arteries in his neck. Stephanie went to the patient's room and saw that he was fully dressed. He had stripped off his hospital bracelet and pulled the IV from his arm. His wife was on the phone, and had tried unsuccessfully to calm him. Stephanie took the phone and listened to the wife explain how her husband sometimes got this way. Exasperated, she asked Stephanie to make sure her husband stayed in the hospital.

Stephanie was just about to approach the patient when she heard the nurse call out to a male intern passing in the hall. "Doctor, you should stay," the nurse told him. "We might need you to make the patient stay." Stephanie grew angry. It was her patient. Why did the nurse assume she couldn't handle the situation? And besides, the patient was eighty. She had no doubt that she could physically control him if needed. She resented the fact that the nurse thought it would take a man to calm this patient down. She walked over to the elderly patient.

"What do you want to do?" she asked him. "You can't go home." She guided him back to the bed and ordered a sedative to call him down. A few minutes later, he was asleep.

Later, she mentioned her frustration to her chief resident. He confirmed what she was beginning to notice—that there were still some female nurses who responded differently to male residents, treating them more like doctors. Nurses were crucial to an intern's life. If you treated them well, if they liked you, they could make life easier. They might update you on multiple patients all at once while they had you on the phone rather than page you incessantly, or they might take verbal orders rather than require you to enter every item into the hospital's computers. Stephanie got along well with most of the nurses. Still, she noticed that sometimes a few looked at her like a student while they treated her male counterparts as doctors.

As Stephanie responded to pages, introducing herself as "Stephanie" and having to take time each call to explain just who she was, she started thinking about what one of her fellow interns had been saying all along. Using the title commanded respect. Introduce yourself as doctor and things moved quicker. She realized she had been wide-eyed and naïve. That night, when the pager sounded, Stephanie picked up the phone and called the number.

"Hello," she said, "this is Dr. Chao from surgery returning a page."

"This is Dr. Barkowski," Rakhi said into the hallway phone.

She had ducked out of the conference room in the Los Angeles hospital. Lunchtime conferences were an important part of an internal medicine intern's education, and just a couple months into her residency, Rakhi did not mind the break in her day. It was a chance to rest her feet and fill up her stomach. She had opted for the vegetarian plate—corn, some mixed vegetables, a roll with butter, and a salad—and had settled into a chair for the lecture on rheumatologic conditions when her pager went off. About forty people sat in the room. They seemed on a constant carousel, leaping up to answer pages on the phone that hung just outside in the hallway, then returning to the room for more of the lecture, which continued without pause. When Rakhi's pager went off, it was her turn to jump.

"Yes, Dr. Barkowski," the nurse began, "your patient's blood pressure is really low." Rakhi asked for the vitals. The nurse explained that the patient's blood pressure was seventy over thirty, and he was diaphoretic, sweating excessively.

Internal medicine was a mind game. Patient histories gave doctors tiny, odd-shaped pieces that, when put together correctly, could clarify a bigger picture. The more experience a doctor had, the quicker the doctor could recognize the cause of a problem. Rakhi's mind raced through her patient's history as she spoke with the nurse. He was a Vietnam veteran a little over sixty years old. He had been Rakhi's patient for several weeks. He was a big man, maybe two hundred pounds. He had come to the hospital for pancreatitis. He once had a cardiac bypass surgery.

Just two months into her residency, Rakhi had learned to think worst-case scenario first, then work from there. The cardiac bypass combined with low blood pressure and sweating all made her think heart attack. Seconds after the nurse gave Rakhi the vitals, Rakhi told her to start an EKG right away and to put oxygen on him. She asked for a portable chest X-ray and told the nurse to put the patient down in his bed in the Trendelenburg position, with his feet resting higher than his head. She wanted to make sure the blood flowed to his brain. Then she dropped the phone and ran.

Rakhi's senior resident—the R3, as a third-year resident is sometimes called—was in the hospital, but Rakhi knew the patient best, having rounded on him for two weeks. She knew that paging the R3 would take valuable time. She would evaluate first, then consult the R3.

It took her about two minutes to run down the two corridors from the conference room to the patient. She took off her white coat at the nurse's station—it would only get in her way—and entered the patient's room. He looked pale. Sweat soaked his sheets. Rakhi tried not to alarm him. She told him she had gotten a call about his blood pressure. She asked him how he was doing. "I don't feel right," he explained. "I feel off."

Rakhi grabbed his hands and squeezed. They were cold, clammy, and sweaty. The chest X-ray was not back yet, but the EKG showed nothing alarming. He said he had no chest pain. She did a quick physical—pressing his belly, listening to his heart—and everything else seemed normal. Maybe it wasn't a heart attack. Her mind went through other possibilities. She remembered giving him a new medication just the day before, Isordil—a drug associated with causing drops in blood pressure. She looked at the record of his blood pressure and saw a dip every couple of hours, correlated with the times he received the medication. That was most likely the cause. She turned to the nurse and asked for saline fluid to help boost his blood pressure. Then she called the R3.

Rakhi explained what she had heard, seen, and how she assessed the patient. "Right now I'm giving him a bolus of fluid, and I stopped the medication," she said. Then she waited for her senior resident's response, nervous for the first time that maybe she had missed something.

"Sounds good," he said.

As the months of internship wore on, the young doctors became more confident in their abilities. One evening past 8 P.M, while Stephanie was on a thoracic surgery rotation, she was assisting the attending and a surgical fellow in the operating room when the fellow got paged. Stephanie enjoyed working with him. He was a friendly guy who wore boots in the hospital and spoke with a thick southern accent. He had been on call the night before and thought this surgery was his last of the day. But thoracic surgery was a consult service, which meant other departments might come calling when they needed assistance. In this case, a woman in the intensive care unit had a ruptured cerebral aneurysm, causing bleeding into her brain. Doctors had attempted to put a catheter called a central line into a major vein to deliver her needed medications, and in the process her lung had collapsed. The problem could be fixed by a chest tube— a tube that could drain fluid, pus, blood, or air from the lung cavity. But they needed someone from thoracic surgery to do it.

The fellow told Stephanie to head upstairs. He told her to get all the supplies they would need and get the patient ready. He would meet her up there. When he did, Stephanie had strapped back the woman's arms to offer clear access to the area just beneath the right armpit where they would insert the tube. The fellow took a Sharpie and drew a black dot on her skin. He told Stephanie that was where she was to insert the tube.

"All right," he said. "Get going. I want to be out of here by 8:25 P.M. You have twelve minutes."

"What do you mean, twelve minutes?" she asked.

"I want to go home," he said, teasing her. "I'm tired. If you don't finish by then, I'm taking your procedure." He smiled at Stephanie. "You've already wasted a minute."

Stephanie moved quickly with the fellow carefully guiding her. She took a long needle and went through the woman's skin, feeling for the bone of the rib. The fellow told her to "hit the rib and march up slowly until you get in." She aimed to scrape the bone gently, then slid the needle up a millimeter at a time until she could just barely slip in above the top of the fourth rib. That way she avoided hitting a neurovascular bundle that could cause significant bleeding or nerve damage. When she thought she was in place, she pulled back on the syringe and saw tiny bubbles in the syringe's fluid, an indication that she had found the intended air pocket. She pinched the needle so it wouldn't move, then threaded a wire through, followed by the catheter.

"Pretty good," the fellow said. "Six minutes."

Stephanie smiled. "I told you I could do it."

When Stephanie came home from her days at the hospital, she was like one of those children's dolls whose eyes close whenever their heads tilt back. As long as she was on her feet, she moved with the same efficiency as she did at the hospital. She breezed through the front door of the East Palo Alto apartment and dropped her bag on the floor. She hurried to the kitchen and grabbed chips or cereal or anything there was to eat. But as soon as she stopped moving and sat on the couch or a chair or in the car if we had to run errands, her eyes began to close. She told me she felt like deadweight. Sometimes, as she napped, she mumbled in her sleep. The patient needs fluids, she muttered. Or someone needed an EKG. The first time I heard this, I tried to reassure her. I had already done it, I said, attempting to ease her back to a peaceful rest. Her brow furrowed. She seemed confused and more agitated. The second time she mentioned work in her sleep, I tried a new approach.

"You already took care of that, sweetie," I whispered.

"Oh, okay," she said, turning over.

Another time, she woke up with a start, terrified that she had slept through an alarm. It took her a moment to realize she had already spent a full day at the hospital. Later, she told me that another resident had dealt with a similar problem by taping a giant sign near the bed one day each week as a reminder that it was a day off.

The problem with Stephanie's schedule, in addition to the long hours, was the lack of predictability. We had found separate apartments within blocks of each other out of respect for her traditional family, though I spent most of my time at her place. But I could never tell what time she would get home from the hospital. And she never knew the four individual days she would get off in a month until that month's rotation began. On the few days off, Stephanie slept much of the day, then woke up disappointed at how many of her free hours had passed.

It was impossible to make plans to see friends or family. Often I went to visit people alone, apologizing for Stephanie's absence. My life was much more predictable. At first, I sat home all day writing my thesis for graduate school. Later, I found a job in the communications department of a local foundation. I drove to work every morning at a little before eight. I returned most days by six. Then I went to her apartment and waited. My resentment grew. Every night was a crapshoot as to what time I would see Stephanie.

Our life together still felt on hold.

7

The Other Important Match
in Their Lives

Michele felt part of her life was on hold, too. A few minutes after midnight, she walked into her hospital's empty waiting room to call Ted. Of all the rooms designated for visitors in Danbury Hospital, this one, on the oncology floor, was the most comfortable. Perhaps it needed to be, giving families of cancer patients a momentary illusion of normalcy. Two chairs and a couch faced a wall unit that attempted to transform the room into a cozy den. Shelves held an eclectic collection of books, a small stereo, and a large Panasonic television. A mural of a fountain and a colorful outdoor garden with life spurting in every direction covered one of the room's walls. Beside it sat an artificial plant.

The television was already on when Michele entered the room. Rock bands and kissing couples flashed across the screen from the Times Square celebration taking place just sixty-five miles south of the hospital. Michele had missed the countdown. She had been sitting at the nurses' station checking charts for new orders, signing her name, the date, and time. Unlike some of the other hallways where moaning and constant commotion filled the air, the oncology floor was quiet, and Michele worked in peace. When she had looked up at the clock to note the time on a chart, she saw it was two minutes to midnight. She signed and dated a few more orders, then got up to call Ted in the privacy of the waiting room.

It was Michele's turn to work the night float. That meant spending New Year's Eve with nurses and cancer patients, while Ted was lucky enough to have the evening off from his hospital. Inside the waiting room, she tried his cell phone. Ted picked up but said he was at a friend's house party. He was leaving soon. He would call her back. So Michele went back to work. She would wait for Ted's call, just as she would wait for him to answer the question she had posed the night before in his apartment.

At first, all the pressure Michele once felt to figure out her future with Ted had dissipated on Match Day with the opening of the envelopes. The artificial deadline passed, and she and Ted were still standing. They had survived the Match. Once she knew that they would be relatively near each other—just an hour and a half apart for year one, and close enough possibly to live together for year two—Michele stopped pushing him to articulate his feelings. They fought less. They enjoyed the final months of medical school. When the lease for her apartment in Manhattan ended several weeks before she could move into the hospital housing in Connecticut, Michele even went with Ted to visit his family in Nebraska and Iowa. They drove from his parents' to his grandmother's house, passing cows along the side of the road and watching the radio display do a full loop while scanning unsuccessfully for channels. It was a bit less exciting than Manhattan, but Michele was glad that Ted brought her home to the family, and that they were spending the time together.

Then residency began. It was the first time in more than two years that she and Ted had not lived down the street from each other. If she was not on call, Michele spent weekday evenings in her one-bedroom apartment on the far side of the hospital parking lot. She dropped on the couch and flipped through television channels, smirking when she came across *Grey's Anatomy,* the show that followed a group of hospital interns. Friends sometimes asked her if this was what her life was really like, but Michele only laughed and wondered where on earth an attending doctor and a resident were making out in the elevators.

Ted had the worse schedule. He worked six days a week whereas, on Michele's first rotation, she had several golden weekends off. There were even days she left the hospital by five in the evening. Some of that had to do with luck—starting her year with emergency medicine meant more shift work than in other rotations. But Michele's program and hospital also seemed an easier place to work. Danbury held only 371 beds, as opposed to the nearly 600 at Ted's hospital. In addition, her hospital tried to place a priority on a pleasant work environment. Life-size posters of smiling nurses populated halls as part of a marketing campaign that announced "I Found It at Danbury," and "A Home Away from Home." The real-life nurses seemed just as nice.

Michele had little problem fitting in. She was gregarious by nature and soon earned a reputation in the hospital as both friendly and competent. At first, everything had felt new, the things she did not know innumerable. She even found herself unsure of how to answer a nurse who asked how much Tylenol

Michele wanted to give a patient she was covering early on one of her first days on the floor. But she was social and vocal and unafraid. If the resident she reported to was hard to find when she had a question, Michele had no problem approaching the attending doctor.

It had not taken long for Michele to grow popular at the hospital, both with the attendings and the staff. While some of her peers seemed ready to check out late in the day, Michele tried never to stand there idle, and offered to help whenever she could. And she did not complain about the work, even though she frequently felt more like a secretary than a doctor.

Much of her day involved checking patient charts, dictating notes, and following through on attendings' orders. While this was not anything unusual for an intern, unlike Rakhi and Stephanie, Michele was not getting to experience her chosen field of medicine. That would need to wait until the next year, when she would begin radiology at Westchester. Still, she was pleased with her match. She loved Danbury Hospital and recognized the perks of working at a wealthy community hospital: orders were processed quickly and without nagging; nurses were helpful and responsive; a pharmacist sat close by to double-check possible drug interactions and doses. And the short walk across the parking lot from home to work meant Michele could sleep relatively late before her 7 A.M. arrival at the hospital.

When she did see Ted, more often than not it was Michele who made the hour-and-a-half drive. She traveled to Long Island if she had a weekend day off and stayed at his apartment. When it really mattered, when her friends at Danbury threw a Halloween party, she made him come north. She wanted to show up to the party in style. She bought Ted a black sheer women's blouse complete with a string across its front. When he arrived, she took eyeliner and drew a mustache above his upper lip. She was sure she had done the perfect job of transforming him into the dedicated farmhand-turned-pirate from *The Princess Bride*. Then she dressed herself as Princess Buttercup. Many of Danbury's residents were foreigners, though, unfamiliar with U.S. movie trivia, leaving Michele to spend much of the party explaining her and Ted's costumes and their relation to each other.

By late December, Michele's frustration was growing again. Her career had progressed. Her relationship had not. One could have blamed the distance and hospital schedules for the lack of time she and Ted had together, but it would have been bearable had Michele any confidence in their future. As the new year approached, she fell back into the pattern of wondering why Ted could not talk about moving in together or marriage. She was tired of waiting for progress in their relationship. For much of her life she had been so focused on her career that now she needed to concentrate on the family aspect. When she eyed the new year on her calendar, Michele thought about her future. She would turn twenty-nine that year. If she could plan everything perfectly, she wanted to become pregnant during her final year of residency, when she would be thirty-two. Ideally, she dreamed about having three children, so that seemed like the time to start.

Plenty of women in Michele's generation delay pregnancy while chasing careers. *The New England Journal of Medicine* noted that the number of first births in the United States among pregnant women between the ages of thirty-five and thirty-nine had increased by 36 percent between 1991 and 2001. But a career in medicine had also focused Michele's attention on the fact that she would reach what had been defined by the medical community as "advanced maternal age" just three years after finishing residency. Even though the threat was still low, pregnancies in women over thirty-five were at greater risk for miscarriages and chromosomal disorders such as Down syndrome. In addition, fertility declined with age.

Michele loved Ted. But she wanted to know she was not wasting her time dating him if he would never end up her husband. Her New Year's resolution, she decided a few days earlier, was to make some decisions about her life that would, as she told Ted, "better my mind and body." For her body, she planned to start exercising—a goal that seemed to make repeat appearances in Michele's annual resolutions. For her mind, she made it a priority to make sure her life and relationship were moving in the right direction. To do that, she needed an answer from Ted.

She had tried to get it the night before, spending that Saturday—her day off—with Ted down on Long Island. She had even warned him about the conversation she wanted to have with him.

"Just so you know, I'm coming down there this weekend, and we're going to talk," she had said. She hoped giving Ted advance notice of the conversation would help. He asked her what she meant.

"A feelings talk, Ted," she said. "You're going to have to think about how you feel."

Michele's frustration did not surprise me. Residency and relationships were turning out to be no great match, as I had been warned, and as I learned firsthand. Stephanie and I struggled to plan dinners together, not knowing what time she would get off on any given night. We either waited to make an easy dinner, maybe throwing pasta in a pot late in the evening, or we ate separately. The biggest problems still stemmed from the lack of predictability. If my cousins invited us to their house a week or two in advance, I thanked them, accepted for myself, and mentioned that Stephanie would need to be a "game-time decision." Some days, I waited at home for hours, unsure when she would leave the operating room. Other nights, I gave up on her and went to the gym in the evening, only to find that she had left the hospital minutes after I put my cell phone in the locker room. I cursed myself for giving up rare time with her, then felt angry at having become a slave to her schedule. Then there were the evenings when Stephanie was on home call and her pager interrupted our conversations every fifteen minutes. I took to teasing her that if that thing beeped one more time I would snatch it and flush it down the toilet. The mental image of the screaming pager swirling out of sight pleased me to no end.

For Michele and Ted, finding time for the relationship to grow had to be even more difficult. The fact that they each kept a resident's schedule at separate hospitals did not help. While they could relate and discuss medical issues on the telephone at night, some of what I imagined to be the perks of a resident-resident relationship were lost on them—no quick coffee together in the hospital cafeteria; no winks or smiles while passing each other in the halls during rounds. And now Michele's original fear that perhaps they had simply been a couple of convenience in medical school was resurfacing.

It was difficult enough to manage one's own life during

residency, let alone try to make a relationship work. A study published in the *Annals of Internal Medicine* four years before Michele, Stephanie, and Rakhi matched made a resident sound like a mental mess. Sixty-one percent of those surveyed for the article described having mood swings and felt that residency made them more cynical. The article spoke to the symptoms of depression and found, not surprisingly, that residents reported sleep disturbance, changes in appetite, and decreased recreational activities. Women fared worse than men. Nearly 40 percent of all female residents reported at least four of the study's symptoms of depression.

A big part of the mental strain for female residents stemmed from concerns about having children. Like their colleagues in other professional fields, women chasing careers in medicine found work dominating their lives at the prime reproductive age. By the time they started residency, most were already older than the average age of a first-time mother in the United States. In addition, many in this generation of doctors had taken what is frequently described as a gap year—time between college and medical school—and entered residency at an older age, thus heightening the tension between career and family.

I had thought about this tension one night at a banquet with Stephanie and her fellow interns just days before they started residency. Each year at that time, Stanford's surgery department put on an elaborate dinner to honor its six outgoing chief residents. They had finally finished the seven-year apprenticeship, and the entire department's physicians and spouses turned out to honor them, with the exception of the unlucky few scheduled to look after the hospital's patients that evening. As dinner was served, attending physicians and residents turned on Power-

Point presentations filled with pictures, and raised their glasses to toast and roast the chiefs. Then the honored guests gave thank-you speeches and smiled in the direction of any family members present.

The new interns were always invited to these dinners as a means of introduction to the department, and Stephanie had asked me to join her. We sat and listened to the speeches. Five out of the six chiefs were men. They seemed proud of their training in the program. But that year, one alluded to a divorce. Another apologized for absence in his partner's life. At another year's dinner, a chief thanked his wife for raising beautiful children as a single parent. I thought of what Dr. Rachlin had said about not wanting to toss away seven years of life, and wondered if the chiefs' families had counted down the days until this moment. Then I looked at our table. Five of the six general surgery residents in Stephanie's class were women—a drastic change from the department's past, and an incredible statistic when compared with the national average of less than 28 percent female surgical residents. None of the women at the table was married. One or two were in relationships. The rest were single. Months later, Stephanie told me about how some other female residents joked about freezing their eggs. That would ensure the opportunity to have children after residency, when they would finally have time for another person in their life.

Regardless of gender, single residents struggled to meet anyone outside the hospital simply because of time constraints. Residents in the early stages of dating nonphysicians often labored to sustain their relationships with people who did not understand their lifestyle. But female residents who wanted children had to worry about the timing of this whole process in a way that their male counterparts did not. As it was, these were people prone to careful advance planning. Their careers had necessitated it. They had passed all the premed requirements long before applying to medical school. They had completed entrance exams more than a year before admittance. In medical school, they contemplated specialties while rotating through a hospital's many departments, then applied to residency programs almost a year in advance. They calculated each step of their career path. So it was no shock that many of these careful planners worried about something not always as controllable—their desired family life—whether they were in relationships or not.

Despite the stigma associated with an expecting resident, both Michele and Rakhi told me that they hoped to become pregnant sometime during residency. Stephanie, on the other hand, wanted to wait. Even though her residency was the longest of the three women, she seemed determined to finish this part of her career before having a child. We had talked about it on the drive back from one of her residency interviews, a few months before the Match. That's when she had told me it was no coincidence that she had gone straight from college to medical school rather than take a year off, as many of our friends did. Stephanie knew that she could not afford to give up a year if she was going to wait to have children. With no time off, she was not as worried. She would be thirty-three upon completion of her surgical residency. Still, she too wanted more than one child. Sometimes she only half joked about how wonderful it would be to have twins because of the efficiency of the whole thing.

Rather than shy away from discussions of pregnancy during residency interviews, Stephanie had taken the opposite approach.

If she met with a male physician, or a female but could not gauge if the doctor had children, she kept her mouth shut. But anytime she met a female physician who volunteered information about her children or who decorated her office with framed photographs of young ones, Stephanie asked questions about balancing a career in surgery and motherhood. Most of the surgical programs she interviewed at included two research years in the middle of the residency. During these years, the young doctors kept a tamer schedule, working out of a lab or office. Some women, she was told, chose to have a child then. But if surgical residents dedicated the first research year to pregnancy— a time when they would not have to be on their feet all day, running the hospital halls—and the second research year to the baby, they still needed to return to the grueling schedule by the time the baby was one year old. That did not sit well with Stephanie. Each time she asked about the best timing, the surgeons she spoke to replied with no definitive answer. The most common answer was that there was no good time to have a child. Plenty of doctors made it work, but no matter when a woman had a child, they told Stephanie, at times it would feel impossible.

As a woman who wanted a family, Stephanie felt it important to have these discussions with the attending doctors and older residents. She had wanted to match at a program where, if for some reason she did have a child during residency, she would not be the first ever to do so. Still, as Stephanie told me of all this, she also said she felt confident that she wanted to wait. She hoped to be there to breastfeed and nurture her baby. She was a modern woman in terms of career, but old-fashioned when it came to thinking about a home life. She struggled to imagine her child running to daddy instead of mommy anytime something was wrong.

Oddly enough, I argued with her. Though I felt unsure about the life that came with Stephanie's chosen career and though we were not even engaged, I often thought about children. While thirty-three did not seem too advanced an age to have a first child in our generation, I knew that a demanding fellowship probably followed Stephanie's residency. And a demanding job followed that. I worried about how long she would want to put off having children. I contradicted myself constantly. After six years of dating, I still waited for our lives to settle before proposing. But a fear of my father's fate also loomed. Friends and family frequently told me that I looked like him, sounded like him, that we had the same mannerisms and same sense of humor. I often worried what else I would inherit. I wanted to make sure I did not wait too long to have children.

When doctors diagnosed my father with cancer the second time, he told me how happy he was to have had fourteen years of remission. It gave him the opportunity to watch his children grow and to appreciate life, he said. Had he died the first time he had cancer, when I was just three years old—the same age he was when his own father died—he was sure I would have had no memories of him.

Once, when I was twelve, I saw him sitting very still on the couch in our living room, and I climbed beside him. He stared ahead and I could tell he was troubled. A flame in the kitchen flickered from a yahrzeit candle—a candle lit on the anniversary of his father's death—and I turned to him.

"Are you sad?" I asked.

He nodded his head.

"But you never knew him," I said.

"I know," he answered.

Had the feelings talk gone the way Michele wanted, she might have felt some resolution by New Year's Eve. She had spent a lot of time bracing for the conversation during her drive down from Danbury to Long Island a couple days earlier, wondering if it would be a defining moment in her relationship with Ted. She cried for some of the drive, listening to Faith Hill on her Volvo's speakers as she turned onto the Cross Island Parkway. The uncertainty of the future ate away at her. She needed some kind of commitment from Ted. Maybe they could talk about finding an apartment together in Manhattan for the following year, since their match results dictated they would work close enough by then, she at Westchester Medical Center, he at Columbia. Or maybe he could just say whether or not he thought they might one day get married. She hated the idea of devoting her entire energy to career, only to learn that she would be on her own. But she also could not stand the thought of losing him.

About twenty-four hours before the ball dropped at Times Square, she and Ted had climbed into the bed in his apartment. They had spent the day together traversing Manhattan with one of Michele's friends who was visiting from out of town, then hitched a ride back to Long Island. The evening wound down and with it departed their one day off. Ted set his alarm for 7 A.M. so he could make Sunday morning rounds.

One day off each week was not enough for Ted. He was an active man, accustomed to adventure and exploration. Even medical school had not slowed him down. He had taken full advantage of the flexibility of a fourth-year medical student's schedule, signing up for a few weeks of language classes in Costa Rica. He was there on the day the rank lists were due and had submitted his from an Internet café, feeling stress-free, away from his classmates and their constant conversations about the Match. He had put New York hospitals at the top of his list because there was still much he wanted to explore. But now his new schedule gave him barely enough time to do laundry or run errands on the one free day each week.

Michele needed to work the next day too, but unlike Ted, she did not have to be at her hospital until the evening. She knew that his alarm would wake her, but took comfort in the fact that she could lounge in bed after he left. She decided she would stay at his place until about 4 P.M. Sundays were usually shorter for Ted, and she figured she would get to see him for a bit before her drive back to Connecticut.

Settled for the night, Michele had turned to Ted. Over the course of their relationship, most of their intimate conversations occurred in bed. Perhaps it was the safest setting for letting your guard down, lying close to someone in the calm of the night. Perhaps it was simply easier to think about dreams and the future before drifting to sleep. Regardless of the reason, once in bed, Michele had decided it was a good time for the talk she had requested on the telephone. She told Ted she wanted to know if the relationship was going somewhere. She asked him his thoughts about their future. She told him she needed some answers from him. Then she waited for a response. Ted had stared back at her. He said he did not have an answer. He said he had not thought about it.

"What do you mean you haven't thought about it?" Michele

asked. She had been asking him to think about it for at least a year. She started to cry. But Ted also looked distraught. He pulled her close, kissed her, and tried to wipe away her tears. Normally Ted was the calm and steady one. Or, when Michele made him angry, he became distant and did not touch her. But this night he had just looked upset in a way she had not seen. Still, he did not say much, and Michele could not stop crying. She felt as if something was crushing her chest. She could not catch her breath.

It was late, and after lying there for some time, Michele told Ted to go to sleep. They would talk about it the next day. Still, she struggled to calm her mind, only drifting off sometime near six in the morning. An hour later, she heard Ted hit the snooze on his alarm, then get up not long after. With him out of bed, she slept a few more hours.

In the morning, while Michele waited for him, she grew calmer and more composed. Ted returned to the apartment not long after noon. They sat on his couch and made a second attempt at the conversation. When Michele envisioned the future, she told him, she saw Ted with her. She saw them raising children together. But, she said, she also deserved to be with someone who wanted to be with her. If he didn't know that he wanted to be with her, then how could she stay in the relationship? How could she wait for him? If he could not see that, she told him, maybe she wasn't the right person for him. It was okay if he did not want to be with her, Michele said. Yes, it would hurt, but she still would rather he told her if that's how he felt. Whatever his decision was, that was fine. But there had to be a decision.

Tears formed in Ted's eyes. He explained to her that he always tried not to think about it. What if she was the right person and he just did not know? he asked. He seemed troubled, and Michele took comfort that maybe now he was finally trying to figure out how he felt. She guessed that he was disappointed with himself for being too scared to make a decision. Even though she had come down to Long Island thinking she needed a definite answer, she backed down. She was not willing to walk away from the relationship if Ted was still trying to make a decision. If she did, she would always wonder if she had left too early.

"Is this something you need a couple days to figure out?" she had asked him.

Ted said yes. So Michele had gotten in her car and driven back to Danbury for her New Year's Eve shift at the hospital, waiting a little longer for some kind of response from Ted.

While Michele and Ted struggled, Rakhi and Scott adjusted nicely to their new life in Los Angeles. Rakhi still felt far from her family—the 340-mile distance meant she needed to use either the rare golden weekend or her schedule's designated vacations to see them—but she was enjoying UCLA. It seemed the perfect fit for her, and she forgot about where it had been on her rank list. Scott proved supportive of her long hours and difficult schedule, too. His reentry into the academic world suddenly had created a more compatible lifestyle for the couple. There was no clear start or stop to his day. He reviewed his economic textbooks and studied much of the time that he was not in class, leaving little time to be frustrated with Rakhi's absence and unpredictable hours. If anything, his life as a student enabled them to spend more time together, driving to and from the university.

Most days, Rakhi and Scott woke up sometime between five and six in the morning. They had only one car and commuted together as much as possible. Scott would grab his backpack and they would drive ten minutes from the apartment to campus. They parted ways in the parking lot at 6:30 A.M. on most mornings but as early as five if Rakhi was working in the medical intensive care unit. Rakhi entered UCLA Medical Center and Scott made his way to the graduate laboratory in Bunche Hall, home of the Economics Department. The campus was frequently deserted at that hour, and the only people Scott saw were ROTC students on their morning run. Once at the Economics Department, he tried to study or review any problem sets before class. Some days, his first class was not until 10 A.M. Other days, it was even later—one or two in the afternoon. Rakhi thought he was crazy for getting there so early, but she liked having his company on the drive in. Then, in the afternoons and early evenings after his classes let out, Scott brought his work to one of the campus libraries.

When Rakhi was close to finishing her day, she called or sent him a text message. Scott would pick up the car. He'd drive to a turnaround just outside the hospital and wait. Sometimes Rakhi could be thirty minutes or even an hour later than she had anticipated. But when that happened, Scott just sat in the car and continued reading. He left the radio on in the background and made the best use of his time. When Rakhi finally came out, they drove home and had dinner.

Neither of them had much time for leisure. Rakhi noticed that they almost never cuddled on the couch in front of the television anymore. Even on Rakhi's rare days off, Scott felt the need to study. He spent so much time working, he joked that he was living a resident's life minus the overnight call. Still, their relationship was strong. On nights when Rakhi had to stay at the hospital, Scott found the Web site UCLA used for hospital staff to send text pages to the doctors, and offered his support. Each time he did, Rakhi heard three beeps from her waist. She pulled out the pager.

"You're a good doctor. I'm glad you're helping people," it read once. "I hope call goes well. Keep up the good work," another time. "Ah, Scotty," Rakhi said to herself. She relaxed whenever she read one of his messages. One night, sometime between midnight and two in the morning, the pager sounded while Rakhi was gloved and gowned. A nurse reached over to Rakhi and pulled out the pager, then read the message out loud: "I hope your night goes well. I'll be thinking of you. I'll see you in the morning."

As the year progressed, Rakhi admitted that if there was one part of her life that felt at all incomplete, it involved her desire to be a mother. She could not help but think about it. Intellectually, she knew it was not logical to have a baby now, but a gut feeling told her otherwise. She described it as instinctual—a deep urge to care for one of her own. She knew she cared for patients all day in the hospital. She made decisions for them. She explained things in layman's terms, taught them about themselves, and held their hands during difficult times. In some ways, she acted like a parent every day. She did not disregard the importance of that experience. But the rewards felt incomplete. When hospital patients got better, they were out of her life.

It was an internal debate for Rakhi. The practical side of her thought there was no logical way to have a baby anytime soon. She reminded herself how difficult it would be as a resident.

One of her fellow colleagues was pregnant and advised against it. "Don't do it in residency," she said. And with Scott in school, and on Rakhi's resident salary, money was tight. Plus, she knew life would get easier in a few years. Internal medicine's residency was the shortest—just three years. But part of her wondered if it would also get easier after the intern year. Regardless of when she and Scott decided to have a baby, she knew she would be ready. She felt that having a baby was a natural part of life. Life marched on, she told friends, even during residency. There was life, she said, beyond the hospital.

Back when I still lived in New York, Ted and I were grabbing a bite to eat one day when he realized just how long Stephanie and I had been dating. "And I'm the one getting pressure?" he teased.

Despite his usual silence on the subject, marriage and family were important to Ted. Too important, he told me, for him to rush into. This was one thing he wanted to make sure of before he committed. He said that Michele kept telling him not to let it worry him if he did not feel 100 percent sure—nobody's ever completely sure, she said—but at the same time, she pressured him for an answer about the future. I could tell Ted felt bad for not having a better idea of what he wanted. But it also seemed that he was not in the same place as Michele. He was in no rush. He once admitted that he probably would not have thought much about these big questions about their future, had Michele not always brought them up. I wondered if there were other issues on his mind, like proving himself as a doctor. The year was frustrating for Ted, not only because he found himself doing what residents referred to as scut work—the boring and menial tasks that made Ted, too, describe his role as that of a secretary—but also because Ted was still waiting to begin his career in anesthesiology. That would not start until the following year, when he would start at the other hospital. During much of this intern year, he felt unsettled, never fully unpacking in the hospital housing. Two boxes filled with picture frames and books sat untouched in his apartment.

About an hour after New Year's Eve changed to New Year's Day, Ted called Michele back at her hospital. They talked briefly, wished each other a happy new year, but did not address the question Michele had raised earlier that day in his apartment.

When Michele related their conversation to me, not long after, I was surprised that she had been willing to give him more time. She had seemed so set on getting an answer out of him. For as long as I had known her, she wanted a concrete sign from Ted. At first, she set her sights on entering the couples' match with him. When that did not happen, she looked to the prospect of living together as the indication of their future. But at other times, she seemed to back off. The same thing had happened on New Year's, and Michele still had no thoughts from Ted about the prospects of a future together. The closest thing to an answer finally came a few weeks later, on a Saturday morning at the end of January.

A morning with no alarm clock was a rare and wonderful thing for a resident, something to be relished and savored for all its sweetness. Michele had driven down to Ted's apartment the night before so that they could share their day off again. They lay in bed in the morning, slowly waking, neither in any hurry to get up. Ted's arms wrapped around Michele and held her. She felt wonderful. "Isn't this so nice?" she said. "Don't you want to do this forever?"

No voice responded. Michele turned to Ted. What was going on in his head? It bothered her that he did not make an effort to communicate his thoughts.

"Is it me?" she asked. "Are you unsure of me? Do you want to be with someone else?" Ted said he did not know what he wanted.

"You can't use that as an answer this time," Michele told him, growing angry. No matter what she said or how she said it, it seemed to Michele that Ted always answered her questions about their relationship with the phrase "I don't know." And yet, she realized, she always made excuses for him in her mind.

Ted told her that maybe being alone would help him figure it out. He suggested they might take a break.

Michele lay there in bed for a moment, withdrawn. She did not want him to touch her. She felt betrayed. Her mind raced. Despite the fact that she had trouble getting him to talk about the future, she always thought they had a great relationship. What was he so unsure of? Why did he not know one way or the other? Then she got up to leave. Ted said he'd talk to her later.

"No," Michele answered. "We're not going to talk." For two and a half years she had been pleading with him to commit to the relationship. He never gave her that, she thought. She got in her car and drove back to Danbury, crying most of the way. She did not know what a break was—wasn't a break just a breakup? "My dad tried to take breaks," she said to Ted when he mentioned it, thinking of her parents' divorce.

For one week, she did not tell anyone. She did not want to

believe it had happened. Part of her was still furious. Part of her blamed herself. And part of her believed there was still a chance. Eventually, she took down the two framed photographs of her and Ted in her bedroom and put them in a box.

8

The Intangible Qualities

I first saw the award when I visited Rakhi and Scott in their Los Angeles apartment. They lived in a university-owned complex designated for UCLA families, about fifteen minutes from where I grew up. On trips to Southern California, I stopped by on occasion to ask Rakhi how she was doing during intern year, or to grab a bite at Tito's Taco's and shoot hoops with Scott if he could take a rare study break. Small children laughed and tottered in the courtyard in front of their home. Inside their two-bedroom apartment, space seemed immense compared to their New York dwellings. They bought a large couch for the living room and set up the second bedroom as a study. Scott's guitar and amplifier stood guard in the corner, as they often had in the old apartment, and diplomas covered the wall above the desk and computer. The award hung in a frame just to the left of Rakhi's medical degree. Beneath blue matting, ornate red and blue letters speckled with gold flakes trumpeted the proclamation:

MATCH DAY

New York Medical College presents the
James Matthew Hagadus, MD Good Physician Award
to Rakhi Barkowski, MD
Selected by the Class of 2006 as one who best exemplifies
those intangible qualities of the "good physician."
May 23, 2006

Rakhi had been thrilled to receive it, particularly because her peers had made the selection. She felt humbled and honored and, I suspect, not entirely surprised. She knew her reputation. Her persona was that of the sweet woman. She was the student, as her peers regularly pointed out, who went into medicine for the right reasons. She projected visions of kindness and concern. As a doctor, they all expected, Rakhi would develop into the model of patience and wisdom, comfort and care. She had an unshakable desire to help people. Whatever those "intangible qualities" were that made up a good physician, Rakhi's classmates knew that she possessed them.

But Rakhi also felt the burden of the award. By the middle of intern year, there were days it pained her to see the award staring back at her. Even though UCLA had turned out to be a good fit, and even though she and Scott had settled into a routine that allowed them to spend their limited free time together on the commute, she admitted feeling worn out by work. There were times when she lost her patience with the hospital staff, she said, only to be disappointed in herself minutes later. The sight of the award upon returning home made her feel worse. On those days, she felt anything but the model physician.

"I feel like it's a big lie," she told me one afternoon when I visited them. "I don't embody that."

I asked her what she meant.

"I notice I get very impatient. I just want to pull my hair out," she said. "I get very irritable with all of this stuff that gets thrown at you. Maybe it's just intern stuff. It's a lot of crap. You have to do paperwork after paperwork."

It was the same paperwork that Ted had complained about, too. He once mentioned that he came into the year hoping to learn as much as he could, but found intern year filled with menial tasks and people barking at him, telling him what to do. The constant orders he had to enter into the charts or the computer wore on him over time.

Rakhi explained to me how ordering a simple set of antibiotics took far too much time and energy, especially when interns were always racing to finish these orders before needing to admit new patients. To order ciprofloxacin, for example, she started by pulling the patient's chart. In the Doctor's Orders section, she made a note to "see the antibiotic order form." Then she signed, dated, and listed her pager number. Next she searched for the actual antibiotic order form, tucked somewhere amid endless other order forms. She noted the name of the drug, the dose, the route ("p.o." for per oral), and frequency ("BID" if the patient was to take it twice daily). Then she signed, dated, and listed her pager number again. Finally, she pulled a green plastic card out of the chart, flagging the folder for the nurse, and put it back on the rack. She knew it sounded like nothing but, when multiplied by what seemed like countless orders on any given day, it felt dreadfully inefficient. Still, that alone would not be so terrible, but the pager constantly interrupted her with questions and requests from the nurses. Eventually, Rakhi stopped sounding like herself when she called the nurses back.

One time, a nurse paged her to say a patient's blood pressure was low. Rakhi asked for the other vitals, but the nurse did not have them. "Next time you call me, you need to evaluate the patient and give me all the vitals," Rakhi scolded. Another time a nurse told her that "Patient 119A has a problem."

"Patient 119A has a name," Rakhi shot back. "You should use it."

Anytime she lost her patience, Rakhi spent the rest of the night beating herself up. "What's wrong with me?" she asked. It was so unlike her to talk to anybody like that. "Why did I do that? What happened to me?" But then it would happen again. And she would feel terrible. *Oh my God,* she thought. *I'm turning into a monster.* She asked Scott to pray for her not to lose her patience.

Almost every resident I spoke with told me similar stories. It was the norm for an overworked intern to get frustrated. What made Rakhi unusual, I suspected, was that she recognized it quickly and held herself to a very high standard. For the most part, her frustration had occurred during one rotation at a county hospital affiliated with her residency program. "I think I'm getting tired," she explained. "I had several days I wanted to run away," she said. "The last thing I wanted to do was be in the hospital."

Friends said that she was being too hard on herself. She was a good doctor. It was understandable that she lost her patience or felt frustrated. That happened to all interns. Rakhi's older residents told her that was nothing new—that February was usually the month when it all got to be too much. It was not just Rakhi. Stephanie's friend Fred, the surgical fellow, told me that he thought that almost every intern reached a breaking point. One night, standing in the hospital's hallway with Stephanie at

11 P.M., Fred could tell she was frustrated. She had spent some of the night struggling to repair a baby's chest tube that kept getting disconnected from the suction source, only to have the patient's family lose faith in her and keep asking why the attending could not do this. Frenzied, and with other patients to see, Stephanie had looked for different pieces of equipment to fix the tube's connection, but could not get it to work. In the hallway, Fred asked her if she wanted to quit.

"No," Stephanie said, then, "Why?"

"Don't worry," Fred told her. "At some point, you're going to want to quit. And if you don't, you're not working hard enough or you're abnormal. At some point, everyone in internship is going to want to quit. When that time comes, please talk to someone."

The residents passed the stories around. They all knew the pressures. One resident knew of an intern who simply left. He was told he did not look too good and that maybe he should go home early. He said that seemed like a good idea. And he chose to never come back.

Somewhere between the pressures and frustrations, though, there were still patients to care for, human beings who were often scared or in pain, who languished in bed all day, awaiting some reassurance from their doctors that they would get through their ailments. The key for interns was to not let the frustrations of a long and trying year get in the way of the empathy they felt for the sick. Becoming a doctor did not just involve knowing what a patient's vitals meant or how to hold a scalpel. There was a human element. To be mature beyond your years, to comfort older patients and families when you were exhausted, overworked, and underconfident—these were not easy things for a first-year doctor to do.

For Rakhi, the challenge was never far from her mind. It was why she had become a physician in the first place. She loved to interact with the patients. Even during the frustrating times, she never forgot the responsibility of caring for other humans with the compassion that led her to the profession in the first place.

Looking at the award on her study wall, it was easy to presume Rakhi was a natural for the medical profession. But she was so deeply empathetic that seeing a person in pain had actually been difficult for her. Once, when Rakhi volunteered at a Santa Monica hospital as a college student, a Spanish-speaking gardener came into the emergency room on a stretcher. He was pale and shivering. He had cut into his leg while using a chain saw, and a flap of mangled calf hung to the side. Rakhi could see layers of muscle and fat. Her job, as a volunteer, was to make patients as comfortable as possible. But when she approached the man, he mumbled, "*Me duele mucho.*" I hurt a lot. There was not much she could do but watch the emergency physician as he cared for the leg. Blood pooled on the blue cloth beneath the patient. Rakhi's adrenaline pumped and she felt in awe both of the human anatomy, as she stared at the inner components of this man's leg, and of the idea of healing the man's wound. She knew she wanted to become a doctor. But when the emergency physician took a syringe and squirted water into the wound to clean it out, the man cringed and moaned. Rakhi felt nauseated. Her stomach tightened. It was not the sight that bothered her as much as his pain. Rakhi couldn't help but to be empathetic toward all living beings.

Even rats. When Rakhi had gone to work in a spinal cord injury lab at her college, she expected to sit at a computer and crunch data. She had not expected to be involved in the study, as the Ph.D. who ran the lab later requested, and to pick up rats and place them on treadmills. Nor had she expected to grow fond of the rats.

Rakhi named them Queenie and Ralphie. Queenie because the female looked so pretty and Ralphie, well, the best way she could explain it was that he just looked like a Ralph. Before the rats made their way to Rakhi, lab attendants had transected their spinal cords between the seventh and eighth segments. They had put gel foam in between the two, then sewed the rats back up. Rakhi's job was to reteach the rats how to walk using a tiny treadmill, and eventually to see the changes in the severed spinal cord. Rakhi lifted the rats and placed them in jackets, which she then attached to a harness on the treadmill. Sometimes she had to tie one leg in the harness too. For thirty minutes, Rakhi had Queenie and Ralphie run or hop on the treadmill. She fed them Froot Loops to keep them happy and watched with joy as they nibbled away at the crunchy rings. Sometimes she turned on the radio— usually light rock—and talked to them while they worked. "How are you doing today?" she greeted them. "Did you have a good night? Did you fight?"

The hard part for Rakhi came at the end of the study. The lab needed to see the way the spinal cord had changed, and the only way to do that was to sacrifice the rats. Someone else in the lab injected the rats with ketamine, a drug often referred to on the streets as "Special K," so that they were anesthetized by the time they came to Rakhi. She asked time and time again if the rats would feel anything and was told no. She felt terrible, but she pushed through. She laid the limp body spread-eagle and cut down the middle with a scalpel. Then she cracked the ribs with her fingers and cut them apart until she could see the rat's heart beating. It was the size of a large grape or hazelnut, with a dark maroon color. The whole process felt wrong to Rakhi. She needed to dissociate. She took a small needle attached to a formaldehyde pump and aimed for the left ventricle. After the heart circulated the chemical throughout the rat's body, she cut off the head, the arms, and the legs, placing each in the red biohazard waste. That left the spinal column for the researchers to study under a microscope. Walking home that night, Rakhi started crying. "I hope this is worth it," she thought. "I hope something comes of this."

She readily admitted that she felt weak when it came to some things. Whenever she was the patient and a nurse or doctor needed to draw some of her blood for tests, she turned her head. She kept her eyes away as the needle entered her vein. She looked anywhere but down as dark red filled the skinny vials. Embarrassed at her reaction, she avoided mentioning her chosen profession during these encounters.

Still, what made Rakhi succeed in becoming a good doctor was her ability to keep the empathy and push past her weaknesses. Once, during the second year of medical school, she confessed a fear to Michele. The medical students had been paired off to practice drawing blood on each other. Rakhi was frightened both of having another inexperienced student poke her in the arm, and of the potential of hurting someone else. When she admitted that to Michele, Michele told Rakhi not to worry. Rakhi could practice on her and stab her as many times as she wanted. Rakhi still looked away when Michele drew her blood, but when it was Rakhi's turn, she felt around cautiously, took one poke, and nailed it. Eventually, she even developed a reputation among her medical school classmates for being especially good at blood draws and IV placement. Still, she didn't like seeing people in pain.

Even by the clinical years of medical school, when she rotated through different services at the hospital, it was hard for Rakhi to stay focused when a patient appeared to be in pain. She'd apologize, then try to ignore the patient as she put in an intravenous line. "You're doing this for their own good, Rakhi," she told herself. "You're not trying to hurt them." Because she knew she was inflicting pain, instinctively Rakhi wanted to stop. She kept repeating those sentences until she convinced herself that the benefit from the IV and antibiotics would far outweigh the pain she had caused.

Rakhi had known that becoming a doctor would mean a lot of challenges, in addition to repaying all of those loans and assuming the enormous responsibility that came with the title. But she wanted to help people, to care for and comfort them. Her peers had congratulated her on choosing internal medicine over the lifestyle specialties—"That's so great," someone said. "They need good doctors like you"—and though she found them condescending, she was always proud of her choice.

During Rakhi's last year of medical school, she had sat through a class in which Dr. Rachlin talked to her medical students about the importance of empathy and compassion. Rachlin showed them the movie *Patch Adams,* in which Robin Williams plays a medical student intent on "treating the patient as well as the disease." *The New Yorker* called the film "embarrassing rubbish" and a "shameless piece of sentimentality," but Rachlin used it to make the point that there might be more to being a doctor than what was traditionally taught in medical school. She asked the students to write down their definition of a doctor and the qualities they wanted to embody as they entered the profession. Rakhi wrote that a doctor was somebody who strove to improve the quality of people's lives—physically, mentally, and emotionally. She wanted to be someone patients would always trust, someone they would find approachable and caring.

A few months before she had graduated medical school and left for UCLA, her father called. He had been having stomach pains and had gone to see his doctor. On the phone, he told Rakhi how his doctor had made him feel better. Just the way the doctor listened and touched his stomach, he explained, comforted him. "I'm so glad you get to do that for people," Rakhi's father said. "And you're going to be great."

Rakhi had hung up the phone feeling focused. *That's right,* she thought. *I'm going to be taking care of other people's parents.*

Ten years earlier, it was my parent who lay dying at UCLA. It was in that hospital that I sat beside my father's bed on a Super Bowl Sunday and watched the television hanging from the ceiling as the Packers hoisted the trophy. The celebration seemed so far away. My father, just inches to my right, drifted in and out of sleep. He was forty-seven years old. Up until six or seven months earlier, he ran a mile every morning and kept careful watch of his cholesterol.

Before he got sick, the man had had more energy than many of his students. He showed up to teach his law class on the first day of baseball season decked out in a New York Mets uniform. He chatted in the hallway after class with any students still interested in talking unless, of course, my sister or I had a game or a play or a school event. On those days, he raced off in his blue Toyota Cressida to meet us. It was the same car he taught me to drive in, a light blue four-door sedan. My father had bought it in Philadelphia to drive across the country and move our family west when I was five years old. Ten years later, when I had my driver's permit, he brought me to the car. He told me to sit behind the wheel, and he climbed into the passenger's seat. I tried to get comfortable, then looked at the dashboard. The odometer marked the car's 99,999 miles. "Drive it around the block," my father told me with a smile. We honked the horn and lifted our hands in triumph as it rolled over to 100,000.

But doctors had found cancer in his abdomen on a July afternoon, and by December, the news was much worse. At first I had only caught the word *brain* through the phone's receiver. I was at a friend's house when my father called to tell me about the latest doctor's visit. Then, like reappearing ink, the five words that preceded it appeared, though their order jumbled in my head. *The* and *in* and *lesions* and *found* and *they.* Then: "They found lesions in the brain."

"What do they mean by lesions?" I had to ask.

"Tumors, Brian," he said.

When I got home minutes later, I found him on the couch by himself, my mother and sister upstairs. He sat very still, wearing the big green ski jacket that we shared, and he stared straight ahead. I wrapped my arms around him and pressed my face into his chest. I clenched my eyes tight, felt him, smelled him, and tried to memorize him.

By the last week of January he was seeing double and hearing ringing in his ears. It took three attempts for him to take his wallet and find his back pocket on the day we left for the hospital. I brought a small compact disc player with us to play music in his room, and occasionally he opened his eyes to join me in the chorus of "The Weight" by The Band. He used to say that, had he not become a law professor, he would have aspired to be either a rock star or a doctor. Hearing him howl along to rock music, even on a good day, left the clear impression that, of the two dreams, only one would have been a viable option. Hardcover copies of *Gray's Anatomy* and *Taber's Cyclopedic Medical Dictionary* sat on his bookshelves at home. He liked to feel informed for his regular visits to the oncologist, a frequent occurrence since his battle with cancer fourteen years earlier. He had always dressed nicely for these encounters, donning a button-down shirt and tie, sometimes even a jacket, out of respect for the profession and with the hope that the doctors would speak to him as a peer. But in the hospital, he ended up dressed in a thin gown draped over a frail body.

The hospital became my entire strange world, those days. I sat with my family inside the lobby, waiting for a neurosurgeon to come and tell us if he had been able to relieve the pressure on the brain. Before the operation, he had described the surgery as opening up the skull and removing some of the fluid that was pushing down on the brain. A family friend had heard of this neurosurgeon. He was a genius, we were told. When I saw the doctor enter the lobby, I expected a success. He was straightforward and to the point, and once again I could not comprehend the words strung together. Minutes later, we were in the intensive care unit. My father lay with his eyes closed and a bandage wrapped around his head. My mother stood at the foot of his bed. Beside her, one of his doctors stood. There was nothing else he could do as a physician, but he stayed there with us. He gently put an arm around my mother as a tear slid down his check. I never forgot the sight.

Sometimes there was nothing a doctor could do but stay and listen.

Despite all that was going on in Michele's personal life, despite her own belief that she was doing only mindless tasks at the hospital, she was growing as a doctor. And work provided an escape for Michele from the drama of her own life. She was the ultimate extrovert, energized by time with her colleagues, and she appreciated the interactions waiting for her each day at the hospital. Alone at home, in the aftermath of Ted's request for a break, she could "fall apart," as she said to me once. She'd occasionally call Ted, maybe even try to see him, though any conversations now felt strained. But at work she was able to remain compassionate and caring, enjoying the social aspect of her job and finding it provided a good distraction.

Michele had grown particularly close to the nurses at Danbury, always chatting with them during the slower moments at the hospital, sometimes going out for a drink with them when they were off duty. Because she was their friend and because she was warm and so approachable, the nurses frequently asked Michele for help, even when the patient was another intern's responsibility. They called her to complain that a patient was not taking his medicine, and Michele would gladly assist. She'd hide the medicine in applesauce or talk to the patient herself, knowing the clout her white coat carried. But among the more pleasant moments were the times she walked into patients' rooms to tell them they could go home. Usually that meant they were in better shape than when they had come in. Usually it meant they were happy and appreciative.

One day, Michele went to discharge someone who had been under her care. The patient was a woman in her seventies with short, thin brown hair. A stroke had left half of her body immobile. She had been admitted to the hospital from a nursing home and now, Michele told her, they would be able to send her back. Michele was getting the papers together so she could go home, she said. She asked if the woman was excited to leave.

"No, not really," the woman said. She could be staying in the hospital and it would make no difference, she told Michele.

Michele was surprised. She had noticed the woman's son, who stopped by every day his mother was in the hospital. He had seemed attentive and caring, even asking Michele questions about his mother's medications. And he frequently came with his father, too, who sat in the corner quietly. But the woman explained that nothing had been the same since she'd had to move to the nursing home. She told Michele about how her husband had dementia and no longer recognized her. A man she had loved for fifty years talked to her now as if she were a stranger passing on the street, she said. Tears came to Michele's eyes. She knew that nothing she could say would make it better. So she sat by the woman's side and took her hand in her own. Together, they sat there.

Amid all the complicated and important decisions and actions, the smallest gestures could make a difference. It was easy to forget that many patients were strangers to the hospital, scared and unsure. The simplest things provided comfort or reminded them that they were surrounded by caring people: telling the patients they were doing better today than the day before; getting some ice for their cracked lips; giving them a tender touch.

On the afternoons in which she was the overnight-call intern, Rakhi frequently glanced at the clock as she sat in the workroom and checked labs. She was constantly aware of the time. She could not get behind. Come 4 P.M., she would need to admit new patients for the night. She wanted everything on her list checked off by that time, so she'd be ready. Rakhi's eyes would often start tearing at about four in the morning. That happened the last few times she had overnight call—it just seemed to be the way her body responded to being so drained. Across the hallway from one of the workrooms was an empty bed for the residents, along with an untouched Velcro dartboard—KNOW WHAT YOU'RE SHOOTING FOR. LIPITOR, it read—but Rakhi rarely expected to lie down; and the only thing most residents were shooting for in the late hours of a call night was a calm evening and morning for them and their patients.

Whenever she got frustrated, she fought to not let that feeling overtake the "good physician" in her. Eventually, she learned to accept the fact that there would be moments of frustration. She forced herself to smile while walking the halls. That physical action alone kept her in a good mood. Interacting with patients came naturally to her. She enjoyed chatting with them, being there for them, and often handed patients a business card so they would be able to remember her name in case they needed anything. And she tried to put them at ease however she could.

One time, while on a rotation at the VA hospital affiliated with UCLA, Rakhi had a particularly cantankerous patient. He was a forty-five-year-old with AIDS, blind in one eye, and weighed about ninety pounds. Rakhi inspected his other eye daily. He was not very happy, and she could understand why. When she came in to ask him how his vision was, he usually replied, "How do you think?" By about the fourth day, his blood counts were going down. He needed a transfusion, and Rakhi brought him a consent form.

"I'll sign only if you do one thing for me," he said. Rakhi was thrown off.

"Well, sure," she answered. "What do you want?"

"I really just want a root beer," he said.

Rakhi was surprised. It seemed like a simple enough request. She smiled and assured him that, as his doctor, she would make sure he got a root beer. He asked if she was serious. Rakhi told him, sure. She'd get him one tomorrow. He gave her a cynical look, catching himself for being hopeful. "Yeah, right," he said. Doctors always say things and never make them happen, he told her. Still, he signed the consent form.

The next morning, Rakhi left her apartment a little early to swing by the 7-11 on her way to the hospital. She bought a plastic bottle of A&W Root Beer and shoved it in the pocket of her white coat. She made her morning rounds, stopping by this patient last. "My vision's just the same, Doc," he grumbled when she entered the room. "Thanks for asking."

Rakhi turned to him. "Before I forget," she said, and pulled out the root beer. He looked stunned. He stammered how he could not believe she remembered. Rakhi smiled.

Just as Rachlin had emphasized compassion to Rakhi's class at New York Medical College, the professors at Stephanie's medical school had required first- and second-year students to attend a course called Foundations of Patient Care. In it, students sometimes had role-playing assignments or practiced talking with people brought in to act as patients, while attending physicians watched and gave them feedback. Still, it was difficult to feel invested in the artificial setup, with an actor playing the part of a patient. But even though Stephanie's role as a resident was often smaller than those she played in the practice sessions, the experience felt distinctly different when real-life patients were involved.

One morning, six family members, an attending doctor, a chief resident, Stephanie, and two medical students all stood in a patient's room. With the full team there, Stephanie's role as the intern was minimal. She listened to her chief and her attending. The patient was a man in his late seventies with a palpable mass bulging from the right side of his abdomen. Although he had moments of lucidity, for most of the time the team was in his room, his eyes remained closed or looked to the side in a sleepy gaze. Rosary beads with a small wood cross lay to the side of his pillow.

The patient had a tumor that involved parts of his kidney, colon, and inferior vena cava. His wound from an earlier biopsy was not healing well, probably because of his poor nutritional status. Several members of the surgical team had spent the previous night trying to explain the issue to the family—that this man was extremely sick, that any surgery might be very hard on him in his condition, and that he would likely end up in the intensive care unit on a ventilator, with the possibility of never coming off. The surgeons wanted to wait until he was stronger in a few weeks, when they might revisit the idea. They also mentioned palliative care as a possibility—treating for comfort, rather than to cure, given the extent of the disease and the poor prognosis. But when an X-ray showed free air in the man's abdomen on this day, indicating that the tumor had led to a rupture somewhere along the patient's bowel, it became a surgical emergency. Untreated, free air could rapidly lead to death. They either needed to operate on him immediately or place him on palliative care. The surgery team needed an answer from the family.

The father had given his oldest son power of attorney, and now the thirty-something son had to lean against the wall, weak from this burden. The rest of the family believed that they should go ahead with the surgery. They did not want to lose their father. But the eldest son hesitated. In a rare moment of lucidity a few days earlier, his father had suggested to him that he did not want surgery. But his father now lay motionless and expressionless. The rest of the family pushed the son to sign for surgery. He asked if his brother could sign in his place. The doctors told him that, unfortunately, it had to be his signature as power of attorney. The son took off his hat and looked up. Tears streamed down his face. He asked the Lord for forgiveness for killing his father. Then he took the consent form from Stephanie's hands and signed.

Stephanie felt terrible for him. The decision would be difficult for anyone to make, let alone with an entire family pressuring him. She was not sure what she would have done in his place. About half an hour later, as Stephanie was back to racing from one task to the next, she saw him in the hallway. His eyes still looked red. Stephanie walked over to him. Her practice sessions had not prepared her for this part, but she felt she had to say something.

"I know you made a very difficult decision," she said, placing her hand on his shoulder. "But it's the tumor that's killing your father. Not you. You are just trying to take care of your dad. I'm sure your father knows that you are trying to help," she said. Then she put her long list with its still-unchecked boxes into her pocket and stood there with him for a moment.

9

Two Rules of Medicine

The long, rectangular box sat on a metal gurney. Wheels rolled on the bottom. White plastic covered the top, wrapped around the entire surface, and hid the box. No handles stemmed from the sides. To move the contraption, hospital orderlies held their gloved hands to the surface and gently pushed. Sometimes they paused outside a room and waited. Usually, they rolled toward the elevator and pressed the down-call button. The apparatus easily passed for a bed or some hospital equipment on the move. Passing patients and families rarely gave it a second look. But Stephanie saw it once or twice every week of her intern year. And each time it made her shiver.

You have a pericardial effusion," the surgical fellow said. It was a technical term for noting that fluid surrounded the woman's heart. Or, to give it a visual, the patient's heart sat in a giant water balloon.

The woman was about fifty years old, though she did not wear it well. She looked thin and frail in the hospital bed. Breast cancer had ravaged her body for years. Doctors labeled her disease as end-stage almost from the start, explaining to her that the cancer had metastasized. On this day, almost four years later, her struggle to breathe had led her to the emergency room. Doctors suspected that the cancer was causing fluid to build up somewhere in her abdomen. They quickly got a CT scan to investigate. But in the top cut of the scan, they happened to see an enlarged heart. That, along with her low blood pressure and fast heart rate, tipped them off to a medical emergency known as a cardiac tamponade. Pressure from the fluid was preventing her heart from beating properly. They inserted a temporary catheter into the space surrounding her heart and drained the fluid. But they knew more would soon accumulate, so the oncology team admitted her to the hospital and called for a surgical consult.

There were many ways a patient could end up under a surgeon's watch outside the operating room. Some patients were admitted to a surgery team's care when there was the possibility of a procedure. Other patients stayed on a surgery team's service while recovering from an operation. And sometimes, even when a different team managed the patient's care, doctors called for a surgical consult, requesting assistance for a specific task. For this woman, the oncology team had requested the cardiothoracic surgeons meet the patient and discuss an operation to drain the fluid. Stephanie was the intern on the team that day.

Inside the woman's room, Stephanie and her more senior surgical fellow explained the operation they wanted to perform. It was called a pericardial window. They would cut off a patch of the membrane that surrounded the heart, leaving a small window in the sack. That way, as her body produced more fluid, it would drain rather than accumulate in a confined space. The procedure would relieve her recent symptoms, they explained, and remove the pressure from the heart.

The woman sat upright in the bed, attentive. She reached for the food tray next to her while the doctors spoke. Stanford Hospital fed its patients well. Often, a couple slices of pineapple, cantaloupe, and honeydew were arranged on a lettuce leaf with a scoop of cottage cheese neatly placed in its center. Stephanie, hungry from not eating all day, watched the woman and her food closely. The woman took a bite. She chewed carefully. Then she spoke.

"You know, I just want to repeat this back to you so I totally understand what we're talking about." The woman spoke slowly and sounded pleasant. She stated everything she had been told. Pericardial effusion. Pericardial window. Draining of the fluid. Stephanie nodded. The woman continued. "So, after this, the oncologist told me they want to do chemotherapy." She took another bite of food. "Well, I'm not sure I want to do this," she said. "The reason being that this is the start of a path that means I'm going to do chemotherapy and I'm going to do other things."

Stephanie interrupted her. "Well, it's not necessarily a package," she said. "We can do the window, but you don't have to do the chemotherapy. They're not all tied together."

The woman said she understood. She explained how, in 2003, when she was diagnosed, she was given a year to live. Four years later, she viewed the extra time as a miracle. But now that doctors were talking about more action, she said she did not want any more procedures. She explained how it seemed to her that doing something, anything, meant starting on a path. She saw two possible paths. "You may think it's crazy," she said, "but one path I do something, the other I wait for a miracle."

A worn, leather-bound black Holy Bible lay on the tray before her, next to the food. The edges of its pages were frayed. A lot of patients brought Bibles into the hospital. Copies were usually well worn, some even with highlighted text. Stephanie had seen plenty during the intern year. She herself believed in God. She even prayed some nights in bed. But residency did not teach physicians to view miracles as standard medical treatment.

As a young doctor, Stephanie, like Michele, had already learned the power of white coat authority—the ability to sway patients to do what the doctors thought best by the way they framed the options, and by how strongly they suggested a pro-cedure or medication or treatment. If this woman had been in her twenties or if her cancer had not metastasized, Stephanie believed it would be irresponsible to accept the woman's an-swer without further discussion. In that situation, she would have worked hard to convince the woman to have surgery, to make it clear to her that surgical intervention would relieve the symptoms and prolong her life. It was a balancing act—always respecting a patient's wishes while making responsible medical decisions.

But Stephanie looked at the woman in front of her and thought for a moment. Surgery might offer this woman a couple more months of life, but it would not save her from the cancer. And, while it might relieve her symptoms, it might also subject her to pain and new discomforts. The woman had seemed calm and rational when she addressed the doctors. She knew what she wanted. It was not easy for a doctor to accept that, with some patients, the disease would ultimately win. Still, Stephanie and the fellow did little to try to change the woman's mind. They asked if she felt certain about the decision.

Yes, the woman said, she was sure.

Death was always present in the hospital. Stephanie told me that there were times when she saw orderlies lift bodies and place them in the long, rectangular covered boxes that rested atop the gurneys. A hospital needed a discreet way to remove deceased patients from the rooms. The bodies needed to make their way down to the morgue, and hospital halls were busy places. You could not just wheel the deceased uncovered, on display for the world. Doing so would not reinforce a hospital's image as a place that could treat even the gravely ill, nor was it very respectful. It was that same logic that had led Stephanie's undergraduate lab instructors to direct her to drape towels over the caged rats she brought up in the elevator from the basement to the upper-floor labs. Why offend people's senses? Everyone knows animal experimentation exists; they just do not want proof. Likewise, everyone knows that people die in the hospital. They just do not want to see it.

Physicians are trained to keep patients alive. In the hospital, they respond to malfunctions that threaten life. Obstructions block the flow of blood. Cells grow at uncontrolled rates. Artery walls swell with plaque. Doctors attend to these problems to save the patients from death. Occasionally one of Stephanie's attending physicians would pass her in the hospital and ask, "How many lives did you save today?" Stephanie smiled. "I don't know about *that*," she usually responded, "but they're all still alive."

Once, while attending a friend's medical school graduation, I heard one of the ceremony's speakers mention that these students would soon assume the physician's role of trying to postpone death. The statement caught me off guard. While I easily associated a doctor's tasks with healing the sick, with treating and even preventing illness, I suppose I never had thought about the ultimate objective inherent in these goals. A lot of doctors would argue other purposes for medicine—stressing quality of life over longevity, and working to relieve suffering—but hearing the speaker phrase it this way made me realize that death was viewed by many as the enemy or as a failure of medicine.

On one hand, postponing death seemed like a worthy goal for the profession and one that I understood. I was afraid of death. I feared the unknown. I feared not getting enough time with my yet-to-be-conceived children. *But you never knew him, I said to my father. I know, he answered.* I recognized that part of this fear might have been influenced by my youth. I was just twenty-eight during Stephanie's intern year, and there was still much that I wanted to experience. But I also knew plenty of people a generation older who feared death, too. Disease and illness and accidents could cut lives short, no matter the age. Doctors diagnosed one of my favorite college professors with colorectal cancer at the age of sixty-eight, just a year before Stephanie's match with Stanford. He lived in California, and I frequently grabbed lunch with him during my trips back to the state. One time, when it seemed the illness was progressing, I got the nerve to ask him how he was coping. He said it was especially hard at night. Lying awake in the dark, he struggled to calm his mind.

At the same time, I recognized that not every person wanted to prolong life. I thought of an older relative who celebrated his ninety-third birthday during Stephanie's intern year. Since his wife's death, he had mentioned to me on two or three occasions how he had lived a good life and was ready for it to end. Despite his age, it felt strange to hear someone talk this way. I wanted to say, "No, you don't really mean that." But of course, he did. It was only the rest of us, his family, who did not want him to leave. We wanted more time with him. Still, he said, he felt ready to die. He had experienced a complete life already. He recognized how this might be hard for me to understand, he said. And he was right. As a young man, I struggled to comprehend someone being ready to die. So I wondered if it might be even harder for young doctors.

As I thought about doctors attempting to postpone death, I realized that they were fighting against inevitability. I asked Stephanie about it one night after she got home from the hospital. "It's a battle between science and nature, and we're always going to lose," she said. She paused for a moment, then added another thought. "But you can change the path; how long that path is, how smooth, and how scenic." It was a lesson Stephanie, Rakhi, and Michele were all learning.

Dr. Rachlin once told me that, although much of medical education focused on keeping patients alive, she also encouraged her students to think of the importance of their actions in times of a patient's death. People remembered how a doctor led them through the terminal events of a loved one, she said. Death was an important part of medicine. She liked to paraphrase some dialogue from the television show *M.A.S.H.* for her students. As I sat in her classroom one day, she recounted it for me. There are two rules of medicine, she said. "Rule number one, patients die." .

"And rule number two?" I asked.

"Rule number two is that doctors cannot change rule number one."

At the beginning of Rakhi's rotation in the intensive care unit, back in November, one of the UCLA second-year residents turned to her in the elevator. He and Rakhi were on their way down to the emergency room to admit a patient to the ICU. He wanted to brace Rakhi. He asked her if she had ever worked on an ICU rotation. Rakhi told him this was her first.

"Just so you know, this is going to be a tough month," he said. "You're going to see a lot of deaths." He told her to keep in mind that these deaths would not mean she was doing a bad job. It was just that these patients were very sick. When the emergency room triaged a patient to UCLA's ICU, it meant the patient was usually in dire shape. Not all of these people would make it out of the hospital's doors.

Hospital work placed doctors in a difficult position. They needed to remain compassionate and understanding people as strangers all around them were experiencing devastation and trying to cope with death. But they also needed to be able to prevent these emotions from interfering with their work. Grieving over every death or internalizing it was not advantageous.

The hardest part for Rakhi, during her month in the ICU, was that a number of her patients were young. Some were in their twenties, thirties, forties—far younger than the patients who seemed ready to die. The younger patients were always full code, meaning they wanted everything possible done to prolong life including, if necessary, CPR, defibrillation to restore the heart's rhythm, and a ventilator to breathe for them. Older patients might not want to be resuscitated, but the younger ones were fighting for a life not yet lived.

One time, as Rakhi stood in the ICU with another intern and discussed a plan for one of the patients, a gathering at the bed five feet in front of her drew her attention. A young man lay still. He looked about twenty-five years old. He was not Rakhi's patient, but she stared at him for a moment, at his full head of hair. The heart monitor to the side showed a slow rhythm. The ICU fellow stood with an elderly woman at the bedside and held her hand. Rakhi had never seen the fellow do that before, and she watched for a moment. Five or six people in all huddled around the bed—family members, Rakhi assumed—their eyes red and swollen. One boy looked about nine or ten years old. Rakhi wondered if he was the man's son, or maybe his younger brother. An elderly man tried to pull the boy closer to the bed. "No, you need to say good-bye," he told him. "You need to get up your strength."

Rakhi felt intrusive. They did not need a stranger watching, she thought to herself. She stood still, said a silent prayer for a few seconds, then tried to continue with her work.

In medical school, anatomy labs allowed students to grow accustomed to cadavers. For the most part, Rakhi had been able to separate her emotions from the task of learning about the body even if, occasionally, hints like the deep groove and tan line on the ring finger of a female hand reminded her that the tools of study before her once lived and breathed.

But medical school could not teach a young doctor everything about death. With death, even with the possibility of death, came a list of tasks and required skills foreign to most people Rakhi's, Stephanie's or, Michele's age. Residents needed to learn how to give bad news to patients. They needed to know how to tell a family when a loved one had died. They had to determine what to do as nurses and relatives and the hospital all waited for them to pronounce a patient dead. They even had to ask patients, who had no reason to imagine the worst-case scenario, to make decisions about how much care they would want in the end.

Whenever Rakhi admitted a patient to the hospital, she needed to inquire about what doctors in the hospital referred to as "code status," so that she knew whether to designate them as DNR (Do Not Resuscitate) and/or DNI (Do Not Intubate). Ordinarily, doctors would attempt to save patients at all costs. If patients did not want the hospital to respond this way should their heart stop beating, if they did not want a tube put down their trachea to allow a ventilator to breathe for their body, they needed to tell their doctors so as to have the DNR/DNI order included in their charts.

It took a while for Rakhi to figure out the best way to approach the topic. It was hard to bring up death with a patient. At first, she did not know exactly how to phrase the question. "Sometimes, when people get admitted to the hospital, things go bad," she said one time. The patient's eyes went wide. "That's not going to happen to you," she said, trying to recover. Later, she laughed at herself as she recounted this awkward attempt. With time, she gained more experience. Before she finished the intern year, she had her part of the conversation fully rehearsed. She waited until she had finished taking the patient's history and conducted her physical examination. By this point, even though she had just met the patient, it felt as if they had established a relationship. It was easier, then, to bring up such a difficult topic. She kept a steady rhythm with her words, a staccato pace.

"Before I step out, I want to ask you this question I ask every-body who comes to the hospital, who gets admitted," she started. "I ask it because I want to respect your beliefs. If something were, God forbid, to happen to you upstairs, if your heart were to stop and we needed to keep you alive artificially, would you be opposed to us doing it?"

Rakhi had practiced her statement a few different ways. She had given thought to whether she wanted to include the words *God forbid*. God was a big part of Rakhi's life, but she under-stood and respected that not everybody shared her view. Still, when she practiced the sentence without these words, it did not feel as natural. For patients who were not clear about what it meant to be kept alive artificially, Rakhi then explained chest compressions and ventilators and codes.

"You mean, you wouldn't do it if I didn't say I wanted it?" some concerned patients asked. Rakhi explained that the default was to always do everything for the patient unless they specified otherwise. "And it's my job to find out what you specify," she said. Almost always, they asked her to do everything possible.

Just as it took a while to feel comfortable bringing up dis-cussions about resuscitation, explaining bad news was an ac-quired skill. One of the older residents reminded Rakhi not to feel responsible. "You didn't do this to them," he said.

Once, on the oncology floor, a patient's daughter asked what was going on with her mother. Another doctor had previously or-dered an MRI, and Rakhi had seen that it confirmed a brain metastasis—the woman's lung cancer had spread to the brain. But the family still did not know. Rakhi told the daughter that the scans were done, but she thought the family should wait for the attending doctor. Rakhi had worried she did not have enough experience to express things correctly.

The next morning, when Rakhi pre-rounded by herself, she stopped by the patient's room. The family had been told the cancer had metastasized, but now they had another question: "What does it mean?"

"It means that it's end-stage," Rakhi said. "There are four stages, and she's at stage four." She stayed to explain that, at this point, the cancer was not curable. There was only palliative care. Rakhi asked them if they knew what that meant. They said no. Without realizing it, Rakhi began speaking as an experienced doctor. She gently explained that it meant they could try to make her more comfortable, but the tumors would always be there.

Rakhi grew more comfortable talking to patients about death as the year progressed. Another patient came in with jaundice. He was a forty-six-year-old man with colon cancer. Recently, the cancer had spread to the liver and was causing an obstruction. A nurse called Rakhi to say the patient's wife was emotional. The nurse wanted to alert Rakhi but planned to call the attending doctor to meet with the wife. Rakhi said that she had gotten to know the patient. She would go in and talk to his wife. Inside, Rakhi introduced herself as the intern on the team. She explained how the cancer had spread. The woman's hands shook as she wiped her tears and blew her nose. But she was grateful for the explanation and information. Rakhi came out feeling that she had done her job.

Rakhi probably saw eleven or twelve deaths during her month in the ICU. Once, she was called to the emergency room to see a patient who had already coded four times. The man was fifty years old, and his family stood by his side. He had a history of vascular disease and stroke. Four times his heart had stopped in the emergency room. Each time, the doctors got it started again, but the amount of time it took—somewhere between four and seven minutes—led Rakhi to suspect he had already suffered extensive brain injury. They moved him upstairs to a bed in the ICU, where an MRI showed the brain damage from lack of oxygen. Still, his family did not want to withdraw care. Rakhi and the other doctors kept him on a plethora of antibiotics and vasopressors—a continuous infusion of medication serving as chemical life support. The patient stayed on Rakhi's service and, two days later, his heart completely stopped again despite all of the medication being pumped through a central line. After seven minutes of trying to get his heart to start again, there was nothing left to do. A nurse asked Rakhi to pronounce the patient dead.

Rakhi went through her mental checklist. She looked at the man's pupils to confirm there was no reaction to light. She pinched his finger and nail to make sure he did not respond to stimuli. Some doctors tested that with what they called a sternal rub, pressing their fists and knuckles hard into the deceased's chest, but Rakhi preferred to pinch the nail. She watched his chest to make sure it did not rise and fall, and placed her stethoscope over his heart to listen for a beat. She held it there for at least thirty seconds, making sure she did not hear a single beat. Then she called out the time of death.

Pronouncing a person dead involved more than just the actual exam. A doctor needed to sign a death certificate listing the cause of death, as well as write a note detailing her final exam. Like most things in the hospital, a death meant a lot of paperwork. Most hospitals had their own versions of what doctors called death packets. The doctor scribbled the date the patient was admitted, the date and hour of death, the cause of death, the name of the nearest relative or friend, and the hour that person was notified. Did the patient have a conservator or public administrator? Was consent for an autopsy obtained? Who was the funeral director designated by the relatives? Was the death note documented in the medical record? Who was the nursing shift supervisor, the intern, the attending physician, the resident on case? Sometimes the death notice might come on a white sheet with two carbon copies. The white page could serve as the medical record, the yellow copy going to vital statistics, and the pink copy staying with the patient's body.

If the family was not already in the room, someone also had to go inform them that their loved one had died. Rakhi walked out with the more senior resident. The patient had been barely alive since coding so many times, and Rakhi suspected the family knew what was coming. The senior resident spoke to the patient's wife. He told her how sorry he was, but they were unable to sustain her husband's blood pressure. Her husband had passed away. The woman started crying, a deep, moaning wail. Her daughter jumped on the room's couch and screamed. "Oh my God. Oh my God," she repeated again and again. Rakhi stood in the corner, quiet. The best thing to do sometimes, she had learned, was to stay still and not say anything.

A thousand thoughts race through a young doctor's mind in those moments, Stephanie once tried to explain to me. "You want to console, but you don't know how. You only met these people days, or even hours, ago. You think, should I say something? Why am I so self-conscious now, of all times, when I should not be thinking of myself? All these thoughts go through your head and you just stand there, still, like a totem pole."

Rakhi did not relish those moments, but she knew it was part of the job. "Willingly or unwillingly, you become a part of these people's memories of death," she told me later.

When a patient was young, death could mean the horror of a life robbed and a battle lost. When a patient was old, it might mean the end of prolonged pain. Patients were often admitted to the hospital for the purpose of preserving life, but it was equally important to recognize when the goals needed to change. While dying was so often a taboo subject in society, Michele saw how direct and open communication about the topic was integral to making sure a patient's wishes were always respected.

One rotation, Michele found herself caring for an elderly man. He was in his late eighties and had been admitted to the hospital by a private physician for fluid in his lungs, raising concerns that he might have a malignancy. In the hospital, the team had ordered blood tests. They took X-rays. They drained the fluid. But they soon recognized that this man's bigger problem was not a possible malignancy, but an exacerbation of his history of heart failure, which now approached end-stage.

In the time this patient had been in the hospital, he had not improved. Rather, he had weakened and deteriorated. His irregular heartbeats blossomed into longer arrhythmias requiring the implantation of a pacemaker inside his chest. He struggled with each breath. Eventually the man's face became hidden behind a mask forming a tight seal over his face, forcing oxygen down his nose.

Yet, Michele was surprised this elderly man remained listed

as full code. And when she and her resident talked to him, they realized he still had expectations that the doctors would be able to cure whatever was causing the fluid buildup. Had his private physician not explained to him that his heart was failing, that he would not get better, and that being listed as full code had consequences? Would he wind up suffering a painful death? If he needed the assistance of a ventilator to breathe for him, he might never be able to come off it.

Whenever private physicians admitted patients, Michele usually saw the doctors visit the hospital in the mornings, before they left for their clinics. But the doctor who cared for this man, who had a relationship with this man, had left on vacation, and the care had been transferred to another physician.

Michele and her resident spoke with one of the attending doctors. They decided they would talk to the family to see if the patient might want to consider having the designation switched to note that he should not be resuscitated or intubated. Michele had spoken with the patient's son and daughter-in-law several times during those two weeks. She knew they, too, were not oblivious to their father's decline. Michele explained to the daughter-in-law that, given the man's current state, perhaps their goals for care should reflect his weakened condition. She explained her team's recommendation.

The conversation had not been as hard as Michele had expected. Having watched the man day after day, she knew he was suffering in his last days. And though she was only the intern, her conversation helped to start the reassessment of this man's goals of care. Michele asked the daughter-in-law to speak to the attending doctors as well. One of the hospital's intensivists, as the physicians who specialized in critical care were known, also went to talk to the patient and his family. The patient and the family all agreed: should his heart stop, should he stop breathing, they did not want him to be resuscitated or intubated. His son and daughter-in-law came into the hospital one more time, not long after, to have a quiet night with their father. The next day, by the time Michele entered the hospital, the man had died, peacefully.

Any patient's death could be hard on a doctor, especially a new doctor who had not yet seen many. But what upset Michele more was how much this man had endured at the end. He had lived a full life. He had not deserved to drag on like this, she thought. She wondered why his private physician had not clearly discussed the situation with the patient and his family sooner.

From watching death approach in so many forms, in so many families, came insights and growth for these new doctors. During the same week that Stephanie saw the elderly woman with the pericardial effusion, she met another patient who also had end-stage cancer. This woman was in her late fifties. Ovarian cancer had spread throughout her body, to the point that chemotherapy would do no good. She still had a head full of salt-and-pepper-colored hair when Stephanie and the surgical fellow entered her room.

The oncology team had called them—another surgical consult—to put a pigtail catheter into the woman's lungs. End-stage cancer frequently caused fluid buildup. In this woman's case, the fluid filled the cavity that surrounded her lungs. The resulting pressure compressed the lungs and made it a struggle to get a full breath. But a pigtail catheter, named for its curly end, could lodge in the chest and, hooked up to a vacuum, drain the fluid and any excess air. Doctors considered it a fairly sim-ple procedure. It was an easy, albeit temporary, fix.

The patient already had one catheter stemming from her chest. While it had helped, her lungs were still somewhat compressed. Oncologists called the surgical team to her room to insert a sec-ond catheter. Stephanie and the fellow carried the pigtail with them. They would be able to perform the procedure right there in her room. But as is the case with any procedure, they needed to explain what they were about to do. They needed to get the pa-tient's signed consent.

The woman smiled when they finished explaining their plan. "I know that my son would want me to do this," she said. "But thank goodness he's not here." She explained that she was tired of having tubes running in and out of her. They could put a tube in, she said, but then what? She did not see the point. It reminded Stephanie of the other patient she had seen that week. The fel-low and Stephanie explained the consequences of not putting the tube in: they told her that she might experience such shortness of breath and feel so uncomfortable at home that she would come back to the hospital.

"You know, at this point, I'm just tired," she said. "Is it okay if I don't do it? I don't want any more lines. I don't want any more tubes. I just want to go home."

"Of course," the fellow told her. "You can decide what you want. But we'll be here if you change your mind."

Later that night, Stephanie thought about the woman. She had noticed a pattern in the hospital. When a patient's family was around, patients often consented to more aggressive treatment. They felt compelled to keep fighting for their families, despite how tired of fighting they might have been. But what did it mean?

Maybe one more month of life for a woman like this, with an incurable disease dominating her every inch? Far too often, terminally sick patients sacrificed for their families, when all they really wanted was to go home.

The next morning, Stephanie made her patient rounds. She stopped by the woman's room to make sure she was still comfortable and that she had not changed her mind. She found the woman thankful and apologetic.

"You were so pleasant yesterday," she told Stephanie. "Thank you for coming to talk to me and trying to help me. But you know, I just don't want another line. I hope that's okay."

Stephanie assured her. Of course that was okay.

"I feel, I just need to say what I want finally," she went on. "Isn't this silly? I was born in an era when you just kind of did as you were told. And it's taken this and me at my age to finally just stand up for myself. I'm not like you young women these days—so smart and strong."

The woman smiled. Stephanie reached out and held her hand. "You're just doing a good job being your own advocate," Stephanie said. "And that's totally okay. That's what we want from you."

Stephanie told the woman that she would continue to visit with her to check on the other tube. Once more, Stephanie reminded the patient that if she changed her mind, then she should say something. But she also knew the woman wanted to go home. The only thing keeping her in the hospital was the first catheter, still hooked up to a vacuum. So the next day, Stephanie disconnected the suction from her catheter. If, after a few hours, an X-ray showed no change to her lung, she could remove the last tube and let the woman go home. The woman said that would be wonderful. Her younger brother was coming to town, and she preferred he not see her in the hospital.

That day at the hospital had been particularly long for Stephanie. She made her rounds on other surgery patients and took care of other orders. When she checked, she saw that the woman's X-ray showed no change in the lung. But the fellow had said, to be safe, they should wait until the next day to remove the tube. It was late in the evening, and she wanted to go home. Still, she pictured the woman in the hospital bed, waiting all day for any news, and she picked up the phone.

"I'm so glad you called," the woman said. "I've been waiting to hear from you."

Stephanie told her that she had just looked at the X-ray. The lung seemed the same. She would leave the tube in one more night, and if it had not changed by the morning, Stephanie would take it out and the woman could go home. "That's wonderful news," the woman said. "Thank you so much."

When Stephanie came home that night, we drove to a nearby coffee shop. It had been weeks since we had gone out anywhere. Stephanie sat still, conserving what little energy remained, I suppose, and sipped a coffee. A year earlier, I would have asked her if coffee so late in the evening might keep her up, but caffeine had little effect on her anymore. Then she told me how the two cancer patients had decided against the procedures. It was interesting, Stephanie explained. These two people were both great advocates for themselves and for what they wanted. It was not something she normally saw. The procedures felt straightforward to Stephanie. For most people, it would have been an easy decision to proceed. "But it's a reminder," she said, "that every small procedure for us is a major decision for them.

"It's just one of these things you tuck away," she said. "I'm becoming more conscious of what we're doing to people. It gives you a better understanding of medicine and your patient."

There was one other insight Stephanie gleaned at some point during the first half of the year as she watched people face death. She shared it with me over dinner one night back in October or November. We had met her family at a local soup and salad place, just within the boundaries of the hospital's short-range pager. Stephanie was on home call that night but figured she could squeeze in a visit and a bite to eat if her parents did not mind a few interruptions. Should the nurses call with an emergency or tell her that a patient needed to be admitted, she would drive ten minutes south on El Camino Real back to the hospital. If they had questions over the phone, she could answer them at the restaurant as easily as at home.

The pager kept beeping at the table that night. Each time, Stephanie flipped open her pink cell phone to dial the hospital. She reached for a pen and took notes on the back side of a restaurant leaflet. Her parents and I watched. The scribbles looked like some sort of architect's drawing. Thin horizontal lines met vertical crosses and ended in diagonals. In the pockets formed by all those crossing lines, she wrote numbers. Nine point nine. One point six with an arrow drawn to two point zero. We all stared in wonder. Later, I asked her about it, and she mumbled something about a patient's elevated creatinine. The move from 1.6 to 2.0 meant abnormal renal function. Something was causing a patient's kidneys to suffer, and she planned to keep an eye on it. But when she got off the phone, she did not say anything other than an apology, and went back to her salad.

Someone at the table asked whether she saw life-and-death cases, and she said that the experience became normal quickly. Death was present in the hospital every day. She had not seen someone die on the operating table, but on the floors—as they called the patient units—she had had many discussions with patients, often having to give bad prognoses. She had taught herself to move on, to treat the next patient, to come home without the weight of loss hanging over her head. Still, she had realized something while watching life in its final stage. She noticed how people nearing death did not speak of all the places they had traveled. They did not talk about jobs or business. The people in the end who were comfortable with death, the ones who were ready to go, were the people who talked about a good family life.

Though that did not surprise me, I made a note. It was an insight that I always wanted to remember.

10

Finding Time for a Life

The alarm clock radio still had another two hours before it would ring.

If I turned it on early, big-band hits would sneak through the static, courtesy of Menlo-Atherton High School's low-powered radio station. Or maybe Scott Simon's friendly drawl would greet me instead, or country or pop or any number of the Bay Area's classic rock favorites, depending on what station had served as the last distraction during the previous evening, as I attempted to stop my mind from racing. But at 7 A.M. on that Saturday morning, the radio alarm—and the phone call it was to remind me to make—were still two hours away. The sun streamed into my East Palo Alto apartment through the window, across a strip of the floor, and finally stopped at the beaten Craigslist couch bracing itself against the far wall of the room. I lay in bed and counted the dots on the ceiling.

The post office worker had said I could call at nine. She would do one last check for me. She promised to scavenge through

Saturday's pile of packages before any of the carriers got to them. If the small box was there, I could come down to the post office and pick it up. I had thanked her profusely when she first made the offer on Friday afternoon. We had become familiar with each other's voices over the last three or four days as I called the local post office each afternoon, trying to figure out why the package was not in my office's mail room or why my colleague Shaka, from downstairs, had not received it, as he did with anything else that was delivered to the office. The package required a signature. It was originally supposed to be mailed to my work address, but with time running out, I was now trying to intercept the package on a Saturday the moment it arrived at the local post office. I had allowed two weeks for it to make its trip from New York, plenty of time considering that my cross-country letters seemed to take only five days. But as each day passed with no sign of the box, I grew more panicked. I called the post office with the tracking number and, every time, was told it would be only another day or two. I did not say what was in the box, only that it had a lot of sentimental value and that I needed it by Saturday.

People had their suspicions at work. Poor Shaka. Each afternoon, after I was sure the mail had arrived, I ran downstairs and fished out whatever letters were in my three-inch slot in the mail room. Then I found Shaka at the front desk. "Nothing, eh?" I asked. He shook his head and said no. I apologized, justified my neurosis by explaining again how it was something important I was having sent here to work so as to be sure somebody would be present to sign for it. He told me he would definitely sign for it and find me as soon as it arrived. I walked back upstairs and reminded myself that I had allowed plenty of time. As long as it arrived by the next Saturday, I was fine. It did me no good until then, I told myself. Upstairs, my friend in a neighboring cubicle smiled every time I returned from the mail room. "What are you up to, Brian?" she asked. I promised her I would tell her later.

After more than a week of checking, I was starting to sweat. I still did not have a backup plan. And I had no flexibility to change the date. Each year, the Stanford surgical interns were assigned three separate weeks of vacation, much like their peers in other residency programs, usually in one-week blocks. Programs often spaced out the weeks so that a resident would get a break from the hospital every three or four months, but depending upon the program, the intern might not have a say in the timing. About two weeks before she began residency, Stephanie had told me of a mass e-mail she received from two of the chief residents, addressed to all of the interns. It noted that they had posted the rotation and vacation schedules on the program's Web site. Each resident's schedule affected the rest. Residents had "vacation coverage" built into their schedules—a month when they spent each week on a different service, covering for the vacationing resident. The e-mail reminded them that the schedule and the vacation dates for the interns were not negotiable.

This particular Saturday, not long after that dinner at which Stephanie mentioned the importance of family, was part of her one week off. She spent the first few days sleeping and the next few catching up with friends and family. Still, she said the week off felt anticlimactic. I assured her I would make her vacation exciting. Really, I said, I would make it worth it.

My last hope was the postal worker. Maybe she had sensed the urgency in my voice that Friday afternoon when she agreed to look for it again the next morning, or maybe she was simply a kind person. But for some reason, that call gave me hope. I looked forward to hearing her voice again. I imagined her telling me, "What luck, it just arrived today." Everything would go exactly as I had planned.

By the time my alarm clock rang, I was already up and showered. I found the phone number on a scrap of paper and dialed. A strange voice picked up. I asked for the postal worker I had been speaking with, and someone placed me on hold. When the woman picked up, I reminded her of my name and the package she had promised to check on for me. Back on hold. Finally I heard her voice again.

"I'm sorry," she said. "But it's still not here."

"Really?"

"Really."

I thanked her and tucked away the cell phone. My heart pounded, my hands twitched. I cursed out loud, then tried to calm myself. It was a good thing Stephanie was spending the morning helping her mother at her house. She would meet me back in East Palo Alto in the afternoon. That left me with a few hours to figure out just what I would do about finding a replacement engagement ring.

For years, Stephanie and I had been teasing each other, testing each other, about getting married. Stephanie would say something ridiculous, and I would mumble, "I can't believe this is the woman I'm going to marry."

"What?" she asked, and I'd pretend I had not said anything at all. "What?" I responded, smiling, trying to look confused. Other times, after she found me entertaining myself with some asinine game, as I was often prone to do, she proclaimed that our children would probably enjoy running into walls with buckets on their heads. "Our what?" I asked. "What?" she responded.

When Stephanie first talked to me about her rank list, she mentioned that Stanford seemed friendlier to the idea of families than some of the other universities. She had met married surgical residents there, even a few with children. And during the first weeks of her internship, she received an e-mail, which she promptly forwarded to me. It came from a social network that appeared to be organized by the wife of one of the more senior residents. The message noted that the network hoped to schedule events throughout the year, including "pizza parties, playgroups, brunches, and wine tasting." Stephanie mentioned to me that she probably would not have time for any of the activities but that maybe I would be interested. I logged onto the group's Yahoo page. There, somebody had posted a list of recommended reading on medical marriages. Ten books were noted. Among the reassuring titles were *Loving the Self-Absorbed: How to Create a More Satisfying Relationship with a Narcissistic Partner* and *Doctors' Marriages: A Look at the Problems and Their Solutions.*

For generations, a doctor's wife was a coveted position in society. Mothers dreamed about their daughters' security if they could only meet that nice, wealthy doctor. But even if a doctor's salary climbed to great heights after he finished residency (and paid off all of the outstanding debt from four years of medical school), doctors and their spouses seemed to have their share of issues. Marriage problems were a popular topic in medicine.

At a spouse component of the fortieth annual meeting of The Society for Thoracic Surgeons, the title of one forum— "Relationship Skills for the Surgical Marriage"—made it seem that between learning about orthotopic tracheal transplantation and surgical management of distal arch aneurysm, a surgeon and spouse could come on over and sign up for a one-day primer on handy relationship skills.

There was no shortage of literature on doctors' marriages. The most amusing pieces were from a few years back, when a headline such as HOW TO SURVIVE YOUR HUSBAND'S RESIDENCY probably did not startle many people. The article, in a 1987 issue of *Resident & Staff Physician,* listed "do's and don'ts" from a surgical fellow's wife. She prefaced her suggestions by reminding readers, "The more of your own creativity you add to each" of the do's and don'ts, "the more likely it will be to charm your husband and make your own life more enjoyable." A resident's wife, she wrote, should learn to function as a single parent and handyman, among other roles, because "the more we can do for ourselves around the house, the more time our husbands can spend enjoying us." She advised wives to be quick and concise about everything they did when their husbands were home, and noted how some wives "use daily updates, much like those used by busy executives' assistants, to keep their husbands informed of family activities, accomplishments, and feelings." Other helpful tips included: "Forget the loans and charge," "Do not expect things to get better just because it's 'next year,'" and "Get a best friend."

A *New England Journal of Medicine* article ten years later addressed medical specialties and divorce. Of five specialties singled out, psychiatry had the highest divorce rate, at 50 percent. Surgery was next, not surprising given the hours and strong personality types of many surgeons. But at 33 percent, it did not sound all that high when compared to the average of 29 percent that the study found among its total pool of physicians. The article noted that female physicians had a higher risk of divorce than male physicians. That hurt our case. High academic achievement in medical school and the death of a parent before graduation appeared to be associated with a lower risk of divorce. I chalked Stephanie up as a high achiever and figured my father's death should count for something.

I quickly passed over *Hippocrates' Handmaidens: Women Married to Physicians* on the recommended reading list, but just in case I thought things were different now that the female was the physician and the male the spouse, the network also included a page labeled "TOP TEN TIPS FOR SURVIVING RESIDENCY—FROM A MALE MEDICAL SPOUSE AND FATHER. In it, the author noted that his "resident wife just doesn't get it" and that "she is so geared up and irritable after being on call there simply isn't enough space in her to think of anyone else."

In an interview about *The Medical Marriage,* the first book on the list, Dr. Wayne Sotile suggested that couples who include a resident physician should think of themselves as in a war zone. "Medical training is not a time for growth in a marriage," he said. "It is a time for personal survival without, one hopes, damaging the relationship."

That seemed to suggest I not propose this year. But Stephanie's medical training would proceed for another six years. And a lack of growth over the next six years would indeed damage the relationship. Life should not have to be put on hold, I decided. Even after Stephanie completed her residency, her career would continue to place more demands on her than most jobs. Pagers would always cry out in our home. Unexpected emergencies would always occur at the hospital. I realized that this was not a one- or two-year bridge. This was not a time for personal survival or a time to wait things out until everything returned to normal. This was a way of life.

I climbed into my old Buick and drove to the nearest mall which, in this case, was next to Stephanie's hospital. On the northwest edge of campus, Stanford had its own shopping center on seventy acres. It was one of the quirks of the school—sparkling stores just a short walk from the medical school. The investment had proved advantageous for the university, bringing high returns for its endowment, but its collection of expensive stores—Tiffany & Co., Neiman Marcus, Louis Vuitton—meant I rarely visited. The only reason I headed there now was that I could think of no other quick options.

My knowledge of jewelry was limited. Stephanie knew that the ring my father had given my mother might be passed down to us, and she thought it beautiful. But both she and my mother had suggested that the setting should be changed before any such use. Since my father's death, my mother had kept the stone in an ornate gold band that she continued to wear but that nobody mistook for an engagement ring. Still, Stephanie had made it clear, when we joked about marriage, that she did not want to go into a store with me to pick out the setting. I found that ridiculous. I asked her if she really needed all these elements of surprise— an unknown ring, a romantic proposal story to tell everyone at work—when we had been together for so many years. Her answer was yes. And yes.

Thankfully, she had left behind a bread crumb. One weekend, while using her laptop, I came across a picture. Stephanie had a number of folders with photographs on the computer's desktop and, while searching a folder for pictures, I noticed a document labeled "ring example." When I clicked on it, a copy of a Web page from an online jeweler popped up. The far right side of the page was cut off, but not before the words *Pavé Diamond Setting*. I made a few notes and printed out the image.

My mother had the stone with her in Los Angeles. Rather than have her mail it to me, I asked her to send her ring to a relative in New York. He would then take it to a jeweler he knew well, who would give me a good deal. The jeweler would remove the stone and put it in a new setting, per the illustration I mailed. Then my relative would mail everything back to me. Somehow it had sounded like a fine plan at the time.

Everything had gone well up until the last step. The stone got to New York. The jeweler made the changes. My relative picked it up and mailed everything back to me. The only thing wrong was our timing. Despite its nonarrival and my realization that I was an idiot, I felt confident that I would eventually get the ring. We had insured the package and it had a tracking number, proof that it was not lost, only late. But that did not help me in the short term. I needed something to place on Stephanie's finger that evening. I had worked hard to set up the romantic proposal she wanted, and I could not postpone my plans.

The thick glass that surrounded the window display case in the first store I tried should have tipped me off that this was not for me, but foolishly I went inside. A saleswoman immediately approached me. I asked her the price on one of the small rings on display. I was in and out of the store in thirty seconds.

Outside, I telephoned Stephanie's sister. After she chastised me for allowing the ring to travel in the mail, we discussed alternatives. Maybe I could use a wedding band, I suggested. Or perhaps I should buy something for the night and return it the next day. Stephanie's sister liked that idea. We both agreed that Stephanie was a thrifty enough person that she would want to return the temporary ring after it served its purpose. I walked over to one of the department stores and found a thin ring with three minuscule diamond embedded in the band.

"You like that one, eh?" an elderly saleswoman said to me. I nodded. She took it out of the case and handed it to me. I wondered if it qualified more as a wedding band than an engagement ring. No large stone protruded from its band. But underneath the display lights, the stones sparkled. The ring seemed tasteful. I took out a slip of paper from my wallet, on which I had scribbled Stephanie's ring size. Stephanie was a size six. This was a seven. Could they resize it for me? Yes, the woman said, but I would need to come back another day to get it. I told her that would not work. I would just take it in its current size. Before I handed over my credit card, I asked about the return policy.

"You know," I quickly clarified, "in case she doesn't like it."

In a letter to the editor of *The Pharos,* a journal of the medical honor society, the former U.S. surgeon general C. Everett Koop wrote about his application to Dr. Barney Brooks for a surgical residency at Vanderbilt in 1942. Koop recounted that "his reply was as clear as it was succinct: 'Dear Koop, You didn't say whether or not you're married. If you are don't answer this letter.'" Koop, who had married his wife, Elizabeth, four years earlier while in medical school, chose the University of Pennsylvania instead.

There was another side to the balance of work and family. As much as I complained that Stephanie was always gone and that our life at home suffered, I knew being in a relationship also put a strain on her training. At the hospital, occasionally Stephanie couldn't help but try to finish up earlier and get home. I asked her about this once, feeling guilty for cutting into her training time. She admitted that, yes, she might not be in such a rush to come home were she not in a serious relationship. Then she laughed, saying she spent enough hours there, and maybe problems at the hospital would be harder to brush off if she did not have someone else.

Still, there were days when Stephanie came home frustrated. After hours of moving fast, of talking quickly and efficiently, she sometimes expected the same at home. If I answered a question in a roundabout way, I could see aggravation in her eyes. If I gave superfluous information, she sometimes interrupted. If I moved too slowly with a chore like cleaning the dishes, she might just opt to take over and do it herself. But after the first few months, this seemed more the exception than the rule. The greatest effect of residency on Stephanie's life away from the hospital simply seemed to be fatigue.

Sometimes I slipped and mentioned how tired I was after work, only to get a piercing stare from Stephanie, who had worked twice as many hours. My colleagues at the foundation liked to tease, when they saw me staying late at the office, that they hired me because they knew my girlfriend was a surgeon, claiming to have accurately predicted that I would work late, having no reason to rush home.

I liked to think of myself as a modern man, strong enough to be with a smart, successful woman. But with each year that I grew more confident about our relationship, I had become less sure of my career. I often felt uncomfortable when, at the hospital, Stephanie's peers asked me what I did for a living. "Working in communications" was vague enough, but inevitably, I would mumble something about being a writer. It usually startled people. They expected the strong female surgeon to be with a lawyer or investment banker or another surgeon. Once, at the hospital, one of Stephanie's fellow interns asked her if she "wore the pants in the family." Stephanie laughed it off, but when she told me the story, it bothered me. Not only would she, in all likelihood, make more money than I would, but also where we would live—what city, how close to the hospital—would always revolve around her.

Still, I tried to remind myself that none of that mattered. I knew I was selfish to be upset by our circumstances, or even by how hard Stephanie was working. I had always felt proud of her decision to dedicate her life to helping other people. "It keeps it interesting," Stephanie liked to tease me about her lifestyle. "I'd be too boring for you otherwise."

With each birthday, with each passing year since college graduation, I had some friends who complained about getting older. I usually smiled when I heard this. Aside from the ridiculous notion that anyone would consider their late twenties old, I pointed out their faulty logic. Did they prefer the alternative? Why fear growing old? I looked forward to it. It beat the alternative. Perhaps, I later realized, that was because I could easily envision my future. I looked forward to growing old with Stephanie. I sometimes teased her that I could see our dentures in matching cups by the sink, me chasing her around the living room with our walkers.

At some point during the previous months, Stephanie and I had discussed potential timing for getting married. There were a few periods each year that she thought a resident would have enough time for a wedding and a short honeymoon, but the best chance, she said, was the period between the intern year and the second year of residency. Because new interns started in her

program a week or so before other residents, the outgoing interns had a little more than a week off in late June before they
began their second year. Of course, I knew that meant I needed
to get my act together with a proposal.

It had been so long since we'd had a social life that at first I had
struggled to think of something Stephanie might like to do for
such a special evening. She loved food—enough that a friend,
watching us in a grocery store, had wisely commented that "a
zest for food is a zest for life." Despite this, we rarely went out to
nice restaurants, either because of time constraints or money.
A more typical meal out involved savoring the $1.50 all-beef
kosher hot dog at Costco, soft drink included. But proposing at
dinner, even at a restaurant a little fancier than our local grocery
store, did not seem unique. I liked better a story I once heard
about a musician who took his future wife for a drive and popped
in a cassette tape. He asked her to listen to a new song he had
been working on and tell him what she thought. In the song, the
lyrics spoke of how he wanted to spend the rest of his life with
her. I also remembered how Scott brought his guitar on the carriage ride with Rakhi, to sing her the song he wrote. Sadly, I had
limited musical ability. Writing Stephanie a song was probably
out of the question unless I wanted to perform it on the kazoo.

With friends and family, I joked about the difficulty of proposing to someone you hardly saw. One relative suggested that
another doctor wheel me into the hospital on a gurney, cloth
draped over my body. When Stephanie walked near, I could pop
up, my outstretched hand holding a ring, and surprise her.

Ultimately, I told Stephanie I had tickets to the opera to celebrate her vacation. She had often mentioned how, as an elemen-

tary school student, her school took a fieldtrip to the pristine War Memorial Opera House in San Francisco. She raved about its towering pillars and sweeping curtains. Whenever the movie *Pretty Woman* appeared on television, when Richard Gere's character flew Julia Roberts's to San Francisco and brought her to the balcony seats at the opera house, Stephanie always smiled and looked swept away along with Roberts's character. But tickets were expensive and often sold out, and Stephanie quickly asked me how I had done this.

"Student rush tickets," I told her.

"Aren't those impossible to buy in advance?" she asked.

"Right," I said, not explaining anything more. Just be prepared to go out Saturday night, I told her.

Now she was doing just that. She had returned after spending the day helping her parents at home and was wrapping a purple scarf around her white turtleneck. I had found my least-wrinkled button-down shirt and grabbed a tie. My sport coat, the same jacket I had owned since college, lay on the couch "just in case it gets cold," I said. While Stephanie put on her makeup in the bathroom, I grabbed the ring box from under the jacket. I could not figure out where to keep it. If it was in my coat pocket, I was sure Stephanie would feel it should she lean into me while watching the performance. If I shoved it into my pants' pocket, I needed to hope she did not brush against me as we walked from the car. I decided to place it in the left pocket and to make a conscious effort to keep Stephanie on my right at all times that night.

Lights flooded the front of the opera house as we pulled up that evening. I knew little about opera, and when I picked up the program for the evening's performance, *Carmen,* I grew nervous. The opera had multiple intermissions. I asked an usher the length of the performance and was told three hours and fifteen minutes. Of course, that included the intermissions. Over three hours, I thought, to try to remain calm.

"How did you get these seats?" Stephanie whispered. I led her up to the first row of the balcony. I said I had my tricks, then smiled and told her to stop asking questions. I walked in front so as to guarantee I would be in the seat to her left, keeping her far away from the bulky ring box. I did not have faith that, as nervous as I was, I would be able to move it to the other pocket. But when Stephanie saw that her seat was on an aisle, she tried to persuade me to switch seats. I had the longer legs, she said. I assured her it was fine.

Then a dreadful thought entered my mind. What if Stephanie needed to be prepared for my post-performance plans? Was it cruel to catch her so completely off guard? "I have one more surprise for you," I said after we took our seats. "Another surprise?" she said, sounding thrilled. I said I'd tell her at the end of the opera.

During each act, I found myself drifting into the story—the beautiful woman pursued by multiple men; soldiers; bullfighters; voices that reverberated throughout the building, throughout my chest—only to recall what I was about to do. Three, four times, I pulled the program close to my eyes in the dark theater, trying to read the synopsis to see how much was left in each act. I scanned how the opera would end—Murder? Really?—and hoped Stephanie would not think this a poor choice of shows.

Intermission. Number one, number two? The evening blurred. Stephanie reached for my hand as we walked to the lobby. She asked me why it was so sweaty. Her own hands had grown dry in the previous months from washing them so vigorously at the hospital every day. Mine, on the other hand, were now dripping. I mumbled something about it being hot and excused myself to go wash my hands. Once again my hands were not the steady tools of my girlfriend's. In the bathroom, I tried to calm down. It was not that I questioned proposing to Stephanie. I felt confident in my decision, and I was pretty sure she would say yes. But I felt nervous about keeping a secret from this woman. I scrubbed the slick sweat off of my palms and returned to Stephanie in the lobby.

We were at the final scene of the final act. I squinted in the dark as I attempted to read the program once more. I put my left hand into my pocket. The ring was still there. On stage, Carmen and Don José battled outside the bullring. They took their final bows. The audience applauded wildly. Then the lights came on and we stood up. Stephanie took my hand and told me it was still sweaty. Once again, unable to think of a better explanation, I commented on how warm it had been inside the theater. Then I reminded her that I still had one surprise left for the evening.

As we walked to the stairway to descend from the opera house's balcony, I could tell Stephanie was still clueless. "We won a contest," I said. She looked skeptical. "Remember when you asked how I got these tickets? Well, we won a contest," I said. She still did not believe me. I told her that the second part of our winnings was waiting downstairs. We were going to be treated to a backstage tour. She told me to stop messing around. At that point, I reached for an envelope tucked in my jacket's pocket.

For some reason, even though the proposal was to be a surprise, I had known Stephanie would enjoy it more if she had at least a few minutes' notice that something big was about to happen. I had spent the night before thinking about what would be a good indicator, just in case, and had come up with the envelope. As I handed it to her, I asked her to look in it for the instructions on who we were supposed to meet for our tour. Now she looked confused. People passed us on both sides, navigating the staircase. I guided Stephanie down the flights as she turned her attention to the envelope. She pulled out the small stack and looked confused. A ticket to a college football game, a television show taping, a concert. "What is all this?" she asked. "I don't understand." It was late already, nearing 11 P.M., and she could not figure out how we had time to attend another event.

"Look at the dates," I said.

Then I saw it click. Her eyes softened as she went through our old ticket stubs again. She was unable to speak, only uttering something that sounded like the beginning of "what" but never reached its final letters. I think I had a representative from almost every year in there: 2000, 2001, 2002 . . . all the way up to the little scrap of paper I had printed that morning with a woman's name. My heart raced. We were almost downstairs. I was almost at my surprise. Had I looked down, I am sure I would have seen pools dripping from my hands, leaving a trail as we walked. When Stephanie got to the final scrap of paper, she managed to speak.

"Who is Marcia?" she asked.

"I'm Marcia," a curly-haired woman said. I could not believe the timing.

The fact that I found Marcia in the first place had a lot to do with luck. That she was such a romantic only made things better. I had shot blindly in the dark and landed the perfect partner for my great surprise.

About two weeks before the big day, I had sent an e-mail blindly to the general Web site address at the opera house. I labeled the e-mail "an odd request" and asked the Webmaster to pass it along to whoever was most appropriate. Then I explained Stephanie's love for the opera and her lack of free time. We would be attending a performance in a few weeks, and I hoped to propose to her there, I wrote. I asked if they provided any tours before or after performances, so that we could walk on the stage when the audience was not present. Then I left my phone number. I knew it was a long shot, but I sent the e-mail anyway. Then I forgot about it.

A week later, Marcia called. She loved the idea. She suggested that I tell Stephanie that I had won a contest that would let us go backstage. Marcia would lead us on a tour and then leave me alone with Stephanie for a few minutes on stage.

"You must be Brian and Stephanie," Marcia said in the lobby. She stood in front of a closed door. Stephanie looked utterly paralyzed now. I had rarely seen her like this. If anything, the months in the hospital had made her able to respond to sudden situations in a calm and efficient manner. But now the surgeon was gone. She looked at me, then back at Marcia, as if to try to figure out how this woman knew our names. "Congratulations on winning the contest," Marcia told her. She tried to engage Stephanie in conversation. She asked if Stephanie had enjoyed the performance. "Yes." As Marcia led us through the door, I could see Stephanie was doing her best to concentrate. She nodded and gave a few "uh-ha"s to Marcia's explanations—"This is the Green Room," and "Standing over there, that is the conductor."

I tried to think of what I would say when we were alone, in what had to be less than a few minutes away. For all of my planning, I had not given much thought to what I would actually say when I asked Stephanie to marry me. Suddenly we were to the side of the stage, peeking from behind wood frames back out at the space we had watched all evening. As if to cue me, Marcia announced the obvious.

"Well, here we are at the stage," she said. Then, turning to Stephanie, "Are you a performer?" Stephanie said no. Well, Marcia explained, maybe you'd like to see what it's like for the performers to be on stage. With that, she walked us out.

Beams of light still flooded the stage. Seville's bullring towered behind us and, ahead, plush orchestra-level seats. A few people milled about in the audience, but for the most part, the opera house was empty. The three of us stood center stage for a moment. Marcia spoke some more, explaining how the video monitor we saw just above the orchestra seats allowed the performers to see the whole stage. Then she said she needed to check on something. She would be back in a minute.

I turned and faced Stephanie. We were both shaking. I grabbed her hands and tried to drop to one knee. Stephanie started sobbing, and I found myself back on my feet reaching to hug her. I told her how much I loved her. I told her that she was my home, that she would always be my home. I asked if she would marry me. Through her tears, she stumbled out two words, then started laughing, the two of us standing onstage in an embrace. "Of course."

I reached into my pocket and pulled out the ring, wondering how I would explain that it was not the one my mother once showed us. But Stephanie was too overwhelmed to notice that, or how in my nervous state I slid it on her wrong hand.

After a few minutes of dabbing her tears, we walked outside to call her mother. I held Stephanie in the cool San Francisco breeze and thought how my father must have had his story right; I was sure I would tell my children that I knew Stephanie was the one from the moment I saw her.

The other ring showed up three days later. The small cardboard package it arrived in wore the signs of a turbulent trip. Multiple stamps and circular postmarks covered its top. Black streaks scuffed a corner; it reminded me of something that had been walked all over and occasionally beaten with a stick. Still, here it was, having survived the journey. I tore it open and gazed at the combination of my family heritage and Stephanie's design. The room's lights glimmered in its surface, and I imagined it on Stephanie's slender hand. During my lunch break, I drove over to the hospital to deliver it.

It was a less than magical moment, by necessity. Stephanie ran outside in her blue scrubs to meet me in the parking lot. She jumped in the car and sat down. I put the ring on her finger—the correct hand this time—and gave her a quick kiss. She smiled at it, told me she loved it. Then the surgeon was up again, running back through the doors of the hospital.

It would always be a tug-of-war. I had come to terms with the idea that I was marrying a woman with a double identity. For the thirty seconds she sat in the car with me, she was the Stephanie I had known for the last six years. But running back into the hospital, she was a woman whose level of responsibility would always be hard for me to relate to, no matter how much I learned from her and from my friends about the culture of becoming a doctor. Stephanie held vulnerable lives in her hands. And those hands could not have anything in their way.

Medicine demanded everything of a person, so I suppose it should not have surprised me that it even demanded the ring. A surgeon's hands needed to be sterile. Even if the gloves could stretch over a ring, the risk of tearing was enough to necessitate that any jewelry come off. That meant Stephanie needed to take off the engagement ring not long after it had gone on. Other doctors faced the same problem. Some pinned their rings to their scrub tops. But Stephanie worried about tossing the top in the hospital hamper without remembering to remove the ring. Instead, she opted to tie it to the drawstring of her scrub pants.

That way, whenever she changed from scrubs to plainclothes, she would be reminded to slip the ring back on her finger as she came home.

11

One Year Down,
the Rest of Their Lives to Go

During the last few months of the intern year, Stephanie and I fell into more of a routine. Often she called me from the car in the evening to let me know she was leaving the hospital. Sometimes she told me about her day—about new procedures she had helped perform or experiences with patients—or asked me about mine. One night in March, as she drove home, she causally mentioned that today had been Match Day.

It was strange to think how a day that had defined our lives one year earlier now belonged to others. Stephanie had not seen the medical students who embraced that morning, envelopes in hand, nor had she heard their screams. She had only shared in whispers along the hospital halls that her surgical program was happy with the new interns it would get in three months. Instead, Match Day—something that once consumed Michele, Rakhi, and Stephanie with months of uncertainty climaxing in a flurry of envelopes and paper, excitement and acceptance—now drifted in the distance practically unnoticed, hidden behind the responsibilities and stresses of their new profession. To the busy and exhausted interns, the third Thursday in March was like any other day in the hospital—making rounds on patients in the morning, filling orders in the afternoon. Its greater significance was simply that it meant there would soon be a new crop of doctors to replace them on the bottom rung of the ladder.

I browsed the newspaper and Web site articles that ran the next day and read how the Match had continued to grow. Almost two hundred more U.S. medical seniors were part of the process in 2007 than in the previous year and the National Resident Matching Program announced that the "number of available residency positions was the highest in Match history."

But what caught my eye more than the statistics were any photos. I saw glimpses into lives altering course, just as ours had: couples opened envelopes together, groups of friends hugged, rejoicing. There was an entirely new batch of doctors on its way to the hospital, and a year behind it, yet another. They would keep coming, the saviors for the sick.

When friends in college first told me they planned to go into medicine, I had applauded them. I viewed the profession as one filled with superhumans. Even after watching my father die, despite the attempts of some of the nation's best doctors, I had viewed medicine and physicians as the magic that provided him with the fourteen years of health that followed his first diagnosis with cancer. Yet as Stephanie, Rakhi, and Michele completed their first year as physicians, it was also now easy for me to see behind the curtain, to know how human doctors were, and to understand the sacrifices they made for this profession.

I felt both respect and resentment for the model of training:

respect because residency seemed to achieve its goals of taking these book-smart medical students and turning them into competent doctors. I saw how much more confident all three of the women were by the end of this one intense year, and could imagine how they would be at the conclusion of residency. If I ever went under the knife, if I ever faced a terrible disease, I would appreciate their years of dedication and experience as I placed my life in their hands. I still viewed medicine as a noble profession, even if I recognized the imperfect humans hiding underneath the superhero white coats. But I also resented how this model pushed everything else in a person's life to the wayside—and sometimes drained young doctors of any feelings except fatigue.

Even as these new doctors gained confidence in their skills by the conclusion of the first year, looking ahead to the stretch of residency that still remained could feel overwhelming, especially on a depleted reserve. Although Stephanie often dodged thinking about the big picture, occasionally it snuck up on her. One day in March, as she and I walked through the parking lot of a McDonald's, her phone rang. Her younger sister was calling to share news of a job offer she had received. Stephanie was the oldest of three siblings. Both her brother and sister worked for investment banks. They worked long hours and made very good money. At one point, toward the end of medical school, Stephanie had reflected that her younger siblings were progressing with their lives while she was still a student. Now, as her sister mentioned the new job offer—a step up from her current level, along with a salary increase—Stephanie congratulated her and told her that was wonderful. But after she hung up, I saw Stephanie's face drop. I asked her what was wrong. She said something about how she guessed her sister was earning three times her own salary;

how she would not make that kind of salary even after seven years of training. I argued with her. A surgeon would make plenty, I said. In fact, her comment made me angry. Eventually, a general surgeon could earn more than $200,000 a year. But that eventuality was hard for Stephanie to recognize, already five years out of college and another six away from the completion of residency.

We continued arguing about it as we got back to the apartment. Tears filled her eyes. She said she was worn out. She was working so hard. She knew it was important for a surgeon to spend these hours and years at the hospital to gain proper training. But while she enjoyed the work and was told she was doing a good job, she also felt stuck. In the time a sixth grader would go through middle school and high school, then pack for college, Stephanie would remain a resident, working long hours, giving up her life, and perhaps peaking at an hourly rate of just over thirteen dollars an hour. This was a hard life, she said, and she did not feel justly compensated.

It was a rare moment for Stephanie. While she had displayed exhaustion and a lack of patience at times during the year, she never complained about her choice. I should have been more understanding. For all I whined about her hours and absence, she— the one actually having to do the work—rarely made a noise. I realized that it wasn't the money as much as the value equated with compensation that bothered her. These young doctors were being worked to the bone, were at the bottom of the hospital hierarchy, and their pay made that all the more clear. The real value in their jobs, I knew, came from the service they provided for others. But telling that to an overworked, overtired doormat did not help.

I reached out to console Stephanie, but my arguing had made

her tense. Later that night, she spoke to her mother, who told her it was okay to cry. Her mother shared some folktale about a group of people on a bus together, something about a woman who got off the bus and decided to walk, making her own path because she knew exactly where she wanted to go. Stephanie, her mother said, just got off the bus earlier than everyone else, that was all. She might have a longer journey, but she knew where she was going. Then her mother reminded her of the good she was doing for the world, of the value in that.

Stephanie calmed down. Her eyes looked swollen after she got off of the phone, but she caught her breath. It was the only time she complained about the money or the number of years of her residency. She tucked her head down and avoided looking at the long road still ahead, the end too far off to see. The next morning, she was back at work.

In the final months of internship, Michele told me how she kept feeling that life was short. Part of this she credited to being surrounded by sick people. Part of it, she joked, might have stemmed from listening to too much of Tim McGraw's album *Live Like You Were Dying*. But the most obvious answer, she said, was that these feelings arose from all the waiting she had done for Ted. Even in the final months of the year, she tried talking to Ted every now and then, and asked to see him if she was down in the city. They chatted about apartment prices and neighborhoods in Manhattan as they looked toward the next year, even going to see a few units together on the Upper West Side. But when they ended up signing leases for two separate apartments—even though the apartments were just blocks away from each other— any thought of living together was finally put to rest for Michele.

As frustrated as Michele was about her personal life, she looked like a confident doctor as the year came to a close. Whereas in the beginning of the year she saw all patients with a resident by her side, when I visited her at Danbury in the final months of her internship, she was frequently on her own. She walked into patients' rooms looking poised and happy, enjoying the banter with even the more combative patients. She talked to them with the care of a teacher, the playfulness of a friend.

"When did the shortness of breath come on?" she asked one elderly lady.

"You know, you ask the same questions day in and day out," the woman responded. Her voice was husky. She was thin but looked as if she had the energy for a fight. She sat upright in her bed, annoyed at being disturbed.

Michele pushed on. She asked if the woman had oxygen at home. "No, and I'm not going to." She asked the last time the woman had smoked a cigarette, and if she wanted a nicotine patch. "Nobody tells this little girl what to do."

"You know," Michele said with a smile, "the other doctor warned me about you." The patient looked pleased. "He did?" she asked, then broke into a big grin. Michele laughed. She was on good terms with the woman now, and each time she returned to the room she would be greeted with teasing, and always compliance.

Michele enjoyed the chatter and bustle of working with other people, but her schedule dictated that she would spend her last two weeks in the hospital on the night float shift—her second time doing so. Night float was never enjoyable for Michele. The hospital felt too quiet. There was nobody to chat with during down moments. Instead, after she checked up on her patients, after she did her scut work, she retreated to the workroom to watch *Grey's Anatomy* episodes online. It was a monotonous existence of going to work, coming home, going to sleep, and coming back to work. Then, after two weeks, night float was over and Michele realized she would never be at this hospital again.

For the past year, Danbury Hospital had been her home and place of work all rolled into one. Even her personal mail had been delivered to one of the hospital rooms, her box on the bottom row along with those of the other preliminary-year residents. She knew that any day now, they would strip her name off the mailbox and replace it with that of a new intern. She would move out of the one-bedroom apartment on the other end of the hospital's parking lot in time for the next rookie doctor to move in. She would bring a U-Haul's worth of furniture and clothes to Manhattan's Upper West Side, where her new home awaited her. One year away from the big city and Michele was returning, glad intern year was over and excited to begin her career in radiology.

Before she left, Danbury held an end-of-the-year awards ceremony. Michele arrived at the hospital's auditorium late and sat down as a speaker handed out a research award. She did not pay much attention to what the speaker said next—something about this being the first year the program had prelims and how glad they were this woman came to their hospital—and then they were calling Michele's name. Her peers, the nurses, and the attendings had voted Michele their intern of the year. Stunned, Michele accepted the plaque.

When I asked her to look back on the year, she reflected that during much of internship she had felt as if she was not offering much, and that a large percentage of her work was secretarial.

She had enjoyed learning but did not find much gratification in the daily tasks. While this seemed true for many interns, I suspected that Michele felt it even more because this was the year she worked outside her chosen field of residency. For Michele, one of the year's benefits was simply that it had enabled her to learn how the hospital functioned. That way, when she began her career as a radiologist the following year, she would have a general understanding of the other departments with which she would work.

Michele also admitted that it was hard for her to give up on Ted completely. She felt she was losing more than just her boyfriend and best friend. In letting go of Ted, she was also letting go of the future she had played out in her mind—of starting a family with him, of their home together, their children together, their life together. Sometimes she would lament to her mother how her friends were getting married and having children and how she had nothing. Her mother reminded her that she had her education; she had the doctorate and she had her career. Nobody could take that away from her. Michele understood what her mother was saying. Eventually she would even come to appreciate it. But at the end of her intern year, she felt disappointed that she did not have a family to go with her career.

Even if the debate continued as to its effects on patient care, many in medicine believed that the eighty-hour-workweek regulations implemented in 2003 had helped residents achieve better balance in their lives. But the big question I kept coming back to was, with this new generation placing a higher priority on lifestyle, were those changes enough to satisfy the new doctors? As much as medical training was steeped in tradition, I wondered if the residency model would be forced to undergo other adjustments in order to avoid the risk of losing the most talented among the new workforce. I suspected that as the new generation moved into leadership positions in medical education, these doctors would implement further change to the residency system.

For one thing, there was a need for more flexibility within residency programs. This was a field that catered to the health of others, and yet among its own, time for going to the dentist or doctor, for sleeping, eating, exercising, and taking care of oneself was almost nonexistent. Furthermore, with medical school and residency programs requiring as many years as they did, it was unrealistic to expect that every female physician would postpone having children until completion of her training. Programs needed to anticipate more pregnancies among residents in the coming years, and address ways to accommodate them.

Residency and fellowship made for a long road, and some in medicine questioned whether doctors who planned to subspecialize might be able to do so earlier in their careers. Becoming a vascular surgeon once meant training for five years in a general surgery residency, plus two research years at many programs, followed by a two-year vascular fellowship, for a total of seven to nine years. But in the last few years, the American Board of Surgery and the accreditation council approved a few integrated vascular surgery residency programs that combined this training into five years. It was not hard to imagine other subspecialties following suit.

Some concerns seemed easier to address than others. Several interns I spoke to mentioned that they did not feel tired on a twenty-four-hour shift because they were constantly moving and keeping busy. Only when they sat in their car for the drive home did exhaustion set in. With extended shifts increasing the likelihood of a resident getting into a car crash, I wondered why more hospitals did not offer taxi vouchers for residents working overnight shifts. I knew of firms in the business world that hired car services for employees who worked especially late at night. If a residency program could find the money, it seemed a worthwhile investment to hire a shuttle or taxi to pick up and drop off the residents working these extended shifts.

But any discussion of residency almost always returned to the issue of hours. In a paper for *The Einstein Journal of Biology and Medicine* in 2003, Bertrand Bell, the doctor who led the Bell Commission, which came up with the eighty-hour workweek, noted that he expected the new work hours would come to be accepted as the norm. And he predicted that perhaps people would next look to the United Kingdom's and European Union's medical workweek, which, Bell wrote, "is even more conducive to patient care and education." Beginning in 2009, he noted, the European Union's workweek for a hospital's trainees would be forty-eight hours.

For many doctors, the debate over hours felt misguided. The supervision of and attention to the teaching of new residents were the more important issues in medical education. I realized that an inherent tension existed in residency. Residents were both employees and students, there for an education. A further reduction in work hours for residents in this country might limit their training and knowledge unless a new education model was also created.

Still, some doctors I spoke with predicted that the focus would continue to revolve around hours and that there would soon be discussions as to whether eighty was still too many. One of the more senior doctors wondered if the new generation's desire for a better lifestyle would manifest in the further reduction of duty hours, hidden behind the idea that long hours hurt patient safety. Others argued that additional studies would indeed show that the first reduction had already helped patient care and resulted in fewer medical errors.

In late March of Stephanie's, Rakhi's, and Michele's intern year, a year after their match, the debate still raged. The chair and three committee members of the House Committee on Energy and Commerce signed a letter requesting that the Department of Health and Human Services work with the Institute of Medicine to determine if long working hours were among the most serious threats to patient safety. In that letter, they cited a report that found medical errors resulting in "adverse events, including death, due to sleep-deprived and overextended medical residents and interns."

By September, the Institute of Medicine had formed a committee to examine medical residents' work schedules and health-care safety, as well as come up with strategies and recommendations regarding both education and quality of care. In welcoming remarks to the committee, the director of the government's Agency for Healthcare Research and Quality noted her excitement about the experts gathered to address what she called one of the preventable causes of error in health care—the extended shifts that residents work. She hoped the committee "could send Congress recommendations that can have an impact on the quality of care across the Nation." The committee was to issue a report sometime in early 2009, and rumors spread among residents in online chat forums and blogs that the report might recommend a further reduction in work hours, possibly even reducing the amount from eighty to fifty-six—a drastic change that others closer to the committee predicted unlikely.

But what would such a change mean for the skills and experience of young doctors? A further reduction in resident work hours could have unintended repercussions for both the hospitals and the residents. Would attending physicians need to increase the number of hours they worked to care for the patients? Would programs need to increase the number of years of residency to make sure trainees finished with enough experience and training? Or might residents simply finish unprepared? An article in the American College of Surgeons' *Surgery News* noted that its own task force on the subject urged the Institute of Medicine committee to evaluate the impact of any further reduction in work hours.

Shortening work hours but extending the number of years of residency seemed implausible, especially as medical education meant assuming a massive debt that could only realistically be paid off with a postresidency salary. Medical school tuition continued to rise, to the point that the annual cost at a public medical school topped $20,000 and at a private one was on the cusp of $40,000. A report from the Association of American Medical Colleges in 2007 showed that student debt had increased, on average, at an annual rate of 6.9 percent over the last six years for a public medical school student to a debt of $120,000; for a private medical school student, the increase was 5.9 percent annually, to a debt of $160,000.

To earn extra cash and help pay off their debts, some residents took to moonlighting after the completion of their intern year—working during any time off, frequently at a hospital unaffiliated with their residency program. Because a moonlighting position might pay anywhere from forty to one hundred dollars an hour, the temptation to work a little more was difficult for a resident in debt to ignore. If doctors found themselves with a weekend off and a desire for more money and more clinical experience moonlighting might look like a good option.

It is hard to know exactly how many residents have the energy to moonlight. An article published in *The American Journal of Emergency Medicine* in 2000 mentioned that 53 percent of emergency medicine residents surveyed said they moonlighted. Another article estimated that the number, for all residents, was closer to 37 percent. In 2003, an unofficial poll in *Virtual Mentor,* published on the American Medical Association's Web site, found 55 percent of respondents claiming to moonlight during residency. But if exhaustion was a problem, moonlighting did not seem a good solution either.

Rakhi would finish out the year in the Cardiac Care Unit as the last intern to take overnight call. She was tired and felt as if she had come to the final leg of a marathon, utterly exhausted and thinking of nothing but the finish line. These last steps seemed to require more effort than the countless others that came before them. It was a Saturday afternoon, and while the other interns finished their year at noon, Rakhi needed to spend one last night in the hospital.

As they left, each of the four other interns in the Cardiac Care Unit signed out to Rakhi, giving her updates on their patients. Then they tried to not flaunt their excitement. Rakhi could tell they were thrilled to leave—there was a giddiness to their last signout. She was bitter at having to stay. At least some tried to downplay their pleasure. A few mentioned that they planned to

go home to relax, rather than detail the exciting plans Rakhi imagined they must have made for the precious week of freedom that
started as soon as they exited the hospital. Of course, Rakhi knew
that any internal medicine interns who did not leave town that
very afternoon would probably find their way to the end-of-the-
year party held that evening at another intern's home—sure to
include drinking and celebrations—while Rakhi would be pre-
siding over heart monitors, medications, and the sick. The others
wished her good luck, told her it would all be over soon, and
bounded out of the unit's doors.

With just one new patient to admit, it ended up being a quiet
night at the hospital. Rakhi was sure a storm of patients and problems would rain down on her, and she stayed awake in anticipation, but the storm never arrived. She briefly lay down on the bed
in the call room but kept her eyes open, chatting with the senior
resident on call, also a woman. The resident mentioned how she
was single and shared her worries about never meeting someone,
what with the demands of this field.

Rakhi was lucky. The year had been difficult and had tested
her patience, but her marriage with Scott was strong and provided support. It helped that Scott had worked so hard that
year, too, that they had practically kept the same hours. It had
allowed her to avoid any feelings of guilt about being at the hospital so much. Scott once mentioned this benefit to me too—
that his work kept him busy enough that he rarely got upset by
Rakhi's hours.

As hard as they both worked that year, there seemed a sense
of security and calmness to their life. All of the uncertainty and
change that had been so present just one year earlier, when they
wondered and fretted over where they would work and live, was

gone. For the entire time of their marriage up until that point, they had needed to move apartments every year. Now, for the first time, they felt settled in their Los Angeles home. One last night at the hospital—just a few hours really—and Rakhi would get to go back to that home to shower, then catch a plane bound for Northern California for vacation and some closure to the year.

A little after five in the morning the new interns arrived. On most days during this last rotation, Rakhi had started in the Cardiac Care Unit at 6:30 in the morning, confident of her speed in seeing patients this late in the year. But as the new interns walked in, she was brought back to twelve months earlier, remembering the fear and excitement and hesitation. She stared at the fresh faces. How well rested they looked. How different they would appear in a year, she thought. She knew her own face advertised the strain of the past twelve months, and she wore glasses over her tired eyes instead of her normal contact lenses. Still, she did not envy the new interns, with all they did not know. She helped them divide up the list—each would take six of the unit's patients—and tried to answer their questions. She heard herself imparting clichés: "Just take it one day at a time." But she also couldn't help herself, admitting to them that it felt so good to be finishing intern year. "You'll be here in no time," she assured them. "Just remember, you're learning a lot, even if you feel you're not."

It was something older residents had told Rakhi throughout the year, and perhaps that was why it came out of her mouth so easily. But as she thought about it now, it was true. So much of medicine was taking a chief complaint and looking for clues, examining the patient history, and putting it all together. She had been so worried in the early months about missing something. But those worries had dissipated as she realized she could identify patients' problems with more and more ease. And she had grown more comfortable interacting with patients and attending doctors. Eventually, she knew, the same thing would happen to the newest class of interns.

Walking out of the hospital that morning, Rakhi felt more tired than ever. But there was also a new sense of satisfaction. *I did it,* she thought. *I climbed a mountain. I made it through the hardest year. And I didn't break down too often.*

When I first set out to understand the life in front of us, the Match seemed foreign and complicated. But one year later, I looked back on it and realized it had ultimately served its purpose well. Perhaps it even taught me a lesson—that not everything was completely within your control in the world of medicine.

Despite the hours, despite the lack of predictability, despite every negative aspect of this lifestyle, one thing made me finally admit that Stephanie had made the right choice in becoming a surgeon: most days, she came home from the hospital pleased with her job. And because of that, we were able to grow excited about our coming wedding.

We tried to plan the big day during any rare moments together. Stephanie's parents said we could get married in their backyard, and my cousin agreed to perform the ceremony. We set the date for the Sunday after Stephanie's last week as an intern, giving us six days for a honeymoon before she would need to be back at the hospital to begin her second year.

The fact that her training as a surgical intern had made Stephanie a model of efficiency didn't hurt the process, either. One female attending, dismayed that Stephanie and I were taking only a few months to plan a wedding, told Stephanie to cut out of clinic early to at least find a wedding dress. Stephanie picked up her mother and went into the first bridal warehouse she saw. By the time she left the store, she had a deal on a gown—veil thrown in for free—and the business card for the owner's brother, the photographer we would hire. Not long thereafter, we went to a local jeweler and bought two plain bands, rings for the ceremony. This time, I kept them close at hand.

The machine that made the hospital identification cards could have been temporarily out of commission on Wednesday, June 20. But the young man and woman adorned in crisp white coats making their way up the hospital's stairs did not need an official badge to designate their status. Their wide eyes and grim expressions gave away the new surgical interns. They would begin work the next morning and had come to check in with Stephanie and the other surgeons to learn about the patients on their rotation.

A pager sounded. "Hear this sound?" one surgical fellow said to the newcomers. "This is tomorrow. Get used to it." The newcomers' heads nodded as the surgeons spoke. They followed the team into patient rooms for afternoon rounds and listened to the lingo and tempo they soon would adopt. Another resident showed them how to use the computer system and how to print reports of patients' vitals. He explained that it might take three or four minutes to print out the reports, and how that would feel in the morning when they had a lot to do. Stephanie added what she had learned early on—that interns should also be prepared to write them out by hand.

Soon a pack of new internal medicine interns in button-down shirts, some with ties, walked through, clearly on a tour of the hospital. The resident leading the group pointed to the side and, as if directing the passengers of an airplane to the Grand Canyon on the right, noted, "Here are the surgical interns." By the nurses' station, someone whispered to the surgical fellow and asked how the group had known. "See how they're smiling?" he responded. "See how our interns look terrified?"

The truth was, all the new interns looked terrified. Their eyes locked in on one another, expressing solidarity, curiosity, and fear without any words. Then the group passed, continuing on its tour. One of Stephanie's peers walked by too and smiled. "The end of an era," he joked, knowing he would be back in the hospital in a matter of days. Still, there was one big difference. When he returned, he would no longer be the "scut monkey," as he called it. Someone else would be fulfilling everyone's orders, racing from nurses' station to nurses' station, chart rack to chart rack.

Stephanie brought the two new interns assigned to her rotation downstairs to the hospital cafeteria. In some ways, it was hard to believe a year had passed since she was in their shoes, a newly matched doctor anxious and nervous and excited to begin intern year. There was still so much she did not know how to do—reason, she figured, for all the years to come in which she would remain a resident. And yet she felt confident in how to be an intern. With these two faces looking to her, she took on a self-assured, comforting air. In the back dining room, where the hospital staff retreated whenever they got a chance to eat, she sat with the newcomers at a table and tried finding some final words of wisdom to impart before their first days as doctors. She passed along advice she had digested over the last year: As an intern, make sure your patients don't die. Know your patients, but don't worry about problem solving, that will come—let the attending doctors figure that out. When you work at night, you're trying to put out fires; get the patients safely to the morning. "It's easy," she said, trying to calm them. "Don't lie. Don't be lazy. And show up."

They went through the patient list together. Stephanie reminded them that they would often be asked when patients could go home. There were five requirements that made this easy to remember, Stephanie instructed. The patients' pain needed to be in control, the patients needed to pass gas, tolerate a diet, have no other major ailments, and have someone able to care for them at home.

The new interns nodded and took notes.

Stephanie reminded them to ask someone if they needed help. Then she got up, finally able to go home herself. The new interns got up as well. They looked at their notes, the new lists in their hands, and divided up who they would see in the morning. Stephanie wished them luck. She watched them for a moment, a small smile on her face.

"We all got through it," she said, "and you will too."

Epilogue

The biggest change in Rakhi's life came during her second year of residency. For a couple days in August, her stomach did not feel right. Her chest burned anytime she drank coffee. She popped antacid tablets throughout the day, but that didn't solve the problem. She wondered if she was stressed, doing too much. The start of the second year had been busy, and though Rakhi loved the added responsibility and the opportunity to teach the younger residents, she was surprised at how her body was now responding. She chatted with another resident while working in the emergency room, casually mentioning how strange it was that she felt this way, since she had never before had acid reflux. The other resident seemed surprised too, then went to get Rakhi something. When the resident returned, Rakhi looked surprised. Still, Rakhi accepted the pregnancy test and tucked it into the bottom right pocket of her white coat, where she kept her wallet and keys. Then she forgot about it.

That evening, at home, Rakhi found it again. Might as well

try it, she figured. She told Scott, then slipped into the bathroom. As soon as liquid hit test, Rakhi was staring at two lines. Positive. She ran and got Scott, and they went to the computer to look up any information attesting to the test's reliability. The next day at her hospital, a blood test confirmed they were having a baby.

Rakhi and Scott were both shocked and excited. It took a little bit of creativity, and a lot of work, but Rakhi figured out a way to shuffle her schedule at the hospital. She moved all of her inpatient rotations to the front of the year and moved her four weeks of vacation to the end. From November until mid-April, she worked six days a week without a vacation, without a break. She spent Christmas Eve and Day, New Year's Eve and Day all at the hospital. By the middle of April, she switched to outpatient rotations, which meant weekends off and fewer hours at work. Still, Rakhi found herself on her feet much of the day and kept working up until the morning she felt the first contractions.

In May, Scott and Rakhi brought their baby girl home. The proud father sent photographs to their friends. In one shot, the baby sleeps on her father's shoulder, her tiny hand spread over the top of his arm. In another, Rakhi holds the swaddled sleeping baby against her body and smiles down at her.

A couple weeks later, as I catch up with Rakhi on the phone, I hear the baby's healthy cries and Rakhi's voice grow tender as she attends to her child.

I ask Rakhi how much time she will get at home before she has to go back to work. She tells me she has eight weeks off— four weeks from the vacation days she saved up, two weeks of maternity leave, and two weeks of sick days. She will ease back into the start of her third and final year of residency on a reading elective, which means seeing outpatients in a clinic for two days each week, along with doing some reading from home. By August, she will go back to the grueling inpatient work at the hospital. That will be her test run, she says, to help her learn how much she can stand to be away from the baby, and to help her decide whether to pursue work in private practice, an academic setting, or a fellowship after residency.

In New York, radiology was everything Michele had hoped it would be—intellectually challenging and stimulating—though there was a steep learning curve. So steep that the hospital would not have a new radiology resident take call for the first six months. Still, Michele finally feels like a real doctor. She raves about her work. She loves interacting with the wide variety of doctors who need her help, and feels she is playing an intricate part in caring for patients without having to do some of the tasks she does not miss from intern year.

"Like what?" I ask.

"Oh, you know, like asking patients if they were able to defecate overnight," she says.

Though she has three more years of residency remaining, she has already begun to think of a postresidency fellowship and is debating further specializing in either pediatric radiology—a return to working with the children she so loves—or women's imaging.

Living in Manhattan and commuting daily to Westchester has not been bad, she tells me. The thirty-five minutes in the morning give her downtime to drink coffee and embrace the day; the ride home allows her to catch up with her mother on the telephone. And the bustle of the city again enables Michele to find distractions easily when she is away from work.

For a while, she and Ted dated again. Then they stopped. This time, when the relationship ended, they did not continue to talk. Five weeks after this final breakup, Michele has gained a new perspective on the matter. "I think I compromised myself a lot these last few years," she tells me. She explains that she had become a person she was not happy with—acting needy and dependent on Ted. "That's not who I want to be."

She still wants a family. She still wants kids. She is still hopeful that she will meet the right person. But she admits that she does not want a man to dictate if she can have a child or not. If she finds herself single as the years continue to pass, she is open to the idea of raising a child on her own. For now, she is thrilled that she has her career.

In June 2007, in Stephanie's parents' backyard, my dear friend Aaron raised a glass of champagne and, to the delight of our friends, toasted "Dr. and Mr. Stephanie Chao."

Two years into her residency, Stephanie still talks shop in her sleep. Most recently, it was something about the spleen and a problem with the appendix. I usually don't respond anymore, confident that she will figure out whatever it is she needs to do.

Like Rakhi and Michele, Stephanie too has considered a postresidency fellowship. She thinks she would like to further specialize, though with another five years of surgical residency to go, she has not settled on anything just yet. Likewise, we have not figured out when the right time to have children will be, though it still seems far in the future and I have grown used to the idea of waiting.

We feel lucky to have each other, even though our life together has its share of stresses. Stephanie's second year has proven equally demanding on her time, with some rotations worse than anything she saw during her first year. In June 2008, she spent a month working the night shift, limiting the time our paths crossed to about thirty minutes every few days and forcing me to sneak into the hospital call room so that I could sit with her for half an hour on our one-year wedding anniversary. Still, Stephanie continues to come home happy most days. She has somehow discovered the ability to get by on even less sleep so that we have time together. And the screams of "pink belly" have returned to our home. To my astonishment, she's even gotten a bit quicker.

Author's Note

This is a work of narrative nonfiction. All of the characters in this book are real, and all are identified by their real names with the exception of Michele and Ted, whose names have been changed to protect their privacy. There are no composite characters.

I conducted interviews with all of the main characters involved during the 2005–2006 academic year, and during their first postgraduate year in 2006–2007. The stories in the book are true, recounted by these people in interviews with the author or witnessed by the author. As with anything, people's memories can differ and occurrences get filtered through the author's perspective. I've tried to capture any scenes as best I can. Dialogue in quotes was either recounted in interviews by someone directly involved in the conversation or heard by the author.

The characters in this book are not intended to represent the entire medical community or the centers at which they work. They are the people whose lives helped educate me as I set out to understand this foreign world.

Acknowledgments

For as many times as I have read the acknowledgment pages in nonfiction books, I still was stunned at how many people's generosity and assistance it took for every stage of this book. I want to express my deep gratitude, first and foremost, to Rakhi, Scott, Michele, and Ted. I could not have written this book without them. Not only were they always helpful, meeting me after long days of school and work, putting up with my endless questions, saving notes and e-mails and tape recordings for me, but they were also so brave in sharing all of their vulnerabilities. When I started working on the book, I mentioned to each one of them that if I ever asked a question that they were uncomfortable answering, just to let me know. It never happened. They never tried to influence what I wrote, and they supported me throughout this project. For all of this, I will always be grateful. I hope the enormous amount of respect I have for each one of them has been conveyed on these pages.

The idea for this book started with an e-mail to a trusted

friend and mentor, the talented author and journalist George Anders. George encouraged me from the start, and I suspect I never would have had the confidence to pursue this book had he not liked the idea. Once I began, George guided and taught me the entire way, serving as a wonderful coach, teacher, reader, and friend.

I have been extremely fortunate to have Aaron Frankel, a friend I consider my brother, by my side for much of my life. I am deeply indebted to him for his help in so many ways at every step of reporting and writing this book. Aaron introduced me to Rakhi, Scott, Michele, and Ted. He helped teach me about medical school and residency, was a constant sounding board and a valuable reader. And, as he has always been, he was there for me as a friend.

Sam Freedman took a chance on me and admitted me to his legendary book seminar class at Columbia University—the most amazing class I have taken. He helped mold my idea for this book and my skills as a journalist, and he continues to be an inspiration.

Steve Schroeder, another one of my most valued mentors and friends, who has taught me so many things in my life and always encouraged me, provided valuable feedback for this book, along with keen insights into the medical world.

Myriam Curet is an inspiration both to her surgical residents at Stanford and to me, and her support and insights made this book possible. She opened many doors for me as I worked on this book, and I've always enjoyed and learned from my conversations with her. I am also very thankful for the support of Paul Costello, in the office of Communication and Public Affairs at the Stanford University School of Medicine. Likewise, I am

Acknowledgments

grateful for the generous help of the people at UCLA and Danbury Hospital.

There are so many other doctors and professors who spent time educating me. A big thank-you to Susan Rachlin for welcoming me into her classroom and talking with me so many times, to Alvin Roth, Sonny Tat, and Fred Tibayan for all that they have taught me, and to Alexis Driggs, who gave me her time despite it not being reflected in this book. Additionally, I am thankful for Barron Lerner's work and writings, which proved helpful for the section on Libby Zion. I would also like to thank the people at NRMP for their hard work every year and for responding to my questions during a busy time. And a thank-you to Dr. Peter Lurie at Public Citizen's Health Research Group for tracking down an old report for me.

During my time working on this book, I received valuable advice from several experienced journalists, including Kevin Cool, Dave Wolman, and Alex Eule. Thank you to each of them. And thank you to Eric Brown, Jack Fischer, and all of my friends at the foundation for being so accommodating and understanding as I disappeared to work on this project.

I try never to miss an opportunity to thank Susan Prager. Thank you to Nick DiGiovanni for kind words and counsel. Thank you, as well, to Marcia Lazar at the SF Opera. Neither Marcia nor I had any idea that the story of the evening would end up in a book when we executed our little plan for Stephanie.

I have been very lucky to get to study at two wonderful universities. A plethora of talented individuals worked at Columbia University's School of the Arts during my time there. Among them, I specifically want to thank Anna Peterson and Leslie T. Sharpe for all of their support. And when I learned I was coming back home to Stanford, one of the first people I grew excited to see was the amazing Bill Woo. You were a wonderful teacher and friend, Bill, and I miss you and our chats by the creek.

I am blessed with a warm and loving family, and I have always gained such strength from them. I want to thank my mother for her love, her amazing attitude, and for always believing in me, and my sister Lisa for her helpful counsel. Dan, Beth, Jeremy, and Laura provided a second home for me while I was in New York and have helped me in more ways than can be recounted here.

I am very fortunate to have an enthusiastic agent in Michael Carlisle, along with his star colleague, Ethan Bassoff. Neither ever gave up on me or this project, and they found the perfect home for it. George Witte, my editor at St. Martin's Press, believed in this from the start and was tireless in making *Match Day* a better book. I am deeply honored to have him as my editor. Likewise, his colleague Terra Gerstner was always helpful and a pleasure.

The final thank-you goes to Stephanie. For sharing every bit of your life, for answering my constant questions, for not caring how strange it might have been to have your boyfriend follow you in public with a notepad, and for always having a smile when I most needed it, thank you.

Notes

Most of the stories and information in this book come from interviews with the main characters. Listed below are some of the additional resources used when referencing statistics, published articles, histories, and other information.

Prologue
3 **more than two thousand cases of orange juice:** Warren E. Leary, "Citing Labels, U.S. Seizes Orange Juice," *New York Times,* April 25, 1991.

4 **about 72 percent of all practicing physicians in the United States were men:** As noted in Table 1: Physicians By Gender, AMA—Women's Physicians Congress (WPC), listing the source as *Physician Characteristics and Distribution in the U.S.,* American Medical Association. Available online at http://www.ama-assn.org/ama/pub/category/12912.html.

1: The Matchmaker
9 **a simple desktop computer running MatchPro software:** The name of the computer program, its approximate speed, and the description of how the monitor displays a series of numbers came from phone interviews

and e-mail correspondence with the National Resident Matching Program
(NRMP) in April and May 2006.

10   **codes on the Match's Web-based "Registration, Rankings, and
Results System."** These codes are listed in the NRMP's *Results and Data*
publications and detailed in the "NRMP Program Code Structure" section of
the report.

10   **until the American Urological Association revealed that there
had been a glitch in the computer system:** Scott Allen, "Tales from
(Mis)Match Day," *Boston Globe,* February 15, 2005.

11   **only spit out 6 or 7 percent of the country's allopathic medical
school seniors:** NRMP's *Results and Data* publication. Table 2: Applicants
in the Matching Program, 2001–2007

13   **weren't paid much, if anything:** see Kenneth M. Ludmerer, *A Time
to Heal: American Medical Education from the Turn of the Century to the Era
of Managed Care* (New York: Oxford University Press, 1999).

13   **fierce competition for the best graduating medical students led to
problems:** Many of the resources for the history of the creation of the Match
and its evolution come from interviews with, and writings by, Professor Alvin
Roth of Harvard University. Roth's work on the subject is insightful and infor-
mative, and several of his papers were helpful. Of particular note is his article
entitled "The Origins, History, and Design of the Resident Match" from *Journal
of American Medical Association* 289, no. 7 (February 19, 2003); and his lecture
to the National Academy of Engineering in 2003 entitled "Matching and Allo-
cation in Medicine and Heath Care." Additional information on Roth's history
and involvement with the Match comes from interviews with Roth in May 2006
and April 2007 at Harvard University, and by phone in November 2007.

16   **an article for *Academic Medicine*:** Kevin Jon Williams, "A Reexam-
ination of the NRMP Matching Algorithm," *Academic Medicine* 70, no. 6
(June 1995).

16 **The Health Research Group:** Public Citizen's Health Research Group and the American Medical Student Association, "Report on Hospital Bias in the National Resident Matching Program," September 1995.

18 **filed an antitrust lawsuit:** Neely Tucker, "Suit Seeks Overhaul of Residency System; Antitrust Action Alleges Conspiracy," *Washington Post,* May 8, 2002; Adam Liptak, "Medical Students Sue Over Residency System," *New York Times,* May 7, 2002.

19 **By 2004, Congress passed legislation:** "SEC. 207. Confirmation of Antitrust Status of Graduate Medical Resident Matching Programs," from the Pension Funding Equity Act of 2004 Public Law 108-218. http://www .govtrack.us/congress/billtext.xpd?bill=h108-3108.

25 **if a candidate didn't interview at enough places:** A helpful comparison of the average length of a rank order list for matched and unmatched applicants can be found on the NRMP's Web site at http://www.nrmp.org/res _match/about_res/impact.html.

2: The R.O.A.D. to Happiness

33–34 **Susan Rachlin:** In addition to Michele's stories about her professor and their meetings, further information stemmed from personal interviews with Susan Rachlin in March, April, and September 2006.

43 **Forty years earlier, the classroom would have looked drastically different:** Statistics on the number of women in medicine then and now come from a number of places, including the AAMC, "Medical Students, Selected Years, 1965–2005," with the enrollment of women in 1966 cited from *Journal of Medical Education* (February 1973); and the more recent years from AAMC's *FACTS—Applicants, Matriculants and Graduates* data, particularly Table 20: Total Graduates by School and Sex, 2002–2006, available online at http://www.aamc.org/data/facts/2006/schoolgrads.htm.

43 **nearly three out of four physicians:** As noted in Table 1: Physicians By Gender, AMA—Women's Physicians Congress (WPC), listing the source

as *Physician Characteristics and Distribution in the U.S.*, American Medical Association. Available online at http://www.ama-assn.org/ama/pub/category/12912.html.

46 **average debt of more than $100,000:** American Medical Association. http://www.ama-assn.org/ama/pub/category/5349.html.

46 **92 percent of senior medical students viewed general surgeons:** E. Ray Dorsey et al., "Influence of Controllable Lifestyle on Recent Trends in Specialty Choice by US Medical Students," *JAMA* 290, no 9. (September 3, 2003).

46 **noted how the Match had seen an increase in the percentage of U.S. students applying to programs in anesthesiology and radiology:** Ibid., "Table 2: US Senior Medical Students Ranking Selected Specialties as Their Top Choice."

46 **One dermatologist noted:** Jack S. Resneck, "The Influence of Controllable Lifestyle on Medical Student Specialty Choice: A Dermatologist's Perspective," *Virtual Mentor* 8, no. 8 (August 2006).

47 **American College of Physicians released a report:** Maggie Fox, "Primary Care About to Collapse, Physicians Warn," *Reuters,* January 30, 2006. This article resulted from the American College of Physicians' report, "The Impending Collapse of Primary Care Medicine and Its Implications for the State of the Nation's Health Care," January 30, 2006.

47 **Articles pointed to a change in priorities:** Among the helpful articles that explored this generation's choices were: Hilary A. Sanfey, "Influences on Medical Student Career Choice: Gender or Generation," *Archives of Surgery* 141, no. 11 (November 2006); and E. Ray Dorsey, "The Influence of Controllable Lifestyle and Sex on the Specialty Choice of Graduating US Medical Students 1996–2003," *Academic Medicine* 80, no. 9 (September 2005). Additionally, Glese Verlander's article, "Female Physicians: Balancing Career and Family," *Academic Psychiatry* 28, no. 4 (winter 2004), proved helpful.

47 **plenty of gender-lopsided residencies:** AMA Table 4: Women Residents By Specialty 2005. Statistics from *JAMA* 296 no. 9 (September 6, 2006). The table is available online at http://www.ama-assn.org/ama/pub/category/12915.html.

4: Match Day

79 **more than nine out of ten:** NRMP's *Results and Data* publication. Table 2: Applicants in the Matching Program, 2001–2007.

85 **According to the agreement that all Match participants signed:** "Match Participation Agreement for Applicants & Programs," Section 6.0, refers to restrictions on persuasion and is available online at http://www.nrmp.org/res_match/policies/map_main.html.

97 **Of the 15,008 graduating U.S. medical students:** NRMP's *Results and Data* publication. Table 2: Applicants in the Matching Program, 2001–2007.

5: Persian Rugs and Getting Pimped

100 **Fred Tibayan:** Personal interviews, April 2007 and February 2008.

103 **equated hand-eye coordination impairment:** Drew Dawson and Kathryn Reid, "Fatigue, Alcohol and Performance Impairment," *Nature* 388 (July 17, 1997), cited in N. J. Taffinder, "Effect of Sleep Deprivation on Surgeons' Dexterity on Laparoscopy Simulator," *Lancet* 352 (October 10, 1998).

103 **self-reported rates of car crashes among residents:** As noted by J. Todd Arnedt et al. in "Neurobehavioral Performance of Residents After Heavy Night Call vs. After Alcohol Ingestion," *JAMA* 294, no. 9 (September 7, 2005); another helpful article on resident work hours and car crashes was Laura Barger et al., "Extended Work Shifts and the Risk of Motor Vehicle Crashes Among Interns," *New England Journal of Medicine* 352, no. 2 (January 13, 2005).

Notes

103   **in a letter to the editor of The** *Journal of the American Medical Association,* **two doctors from Irvine:** James Robert Wendt and Lester J. Yen, "The Resident by Moonlight: A Misguided Missile," *JAMA* 259, no. 1 (January 1, 1998).

104   **just over $43,000:** AAMC Survey of Housestaff Stipends, Benefits, and Funding 2006 survey. Available online at www.aamc.org/data/housestaff.

104   **a CBS MarketWatch columnist in 2003:** "Ten Most Underpaid Jobs in the U.S. Commentary: Most Require Skill, Courage and Heart," Chris Pummer, *CBS MarketWatch,* November 13, 2003.

105   **Sidney Zion:** Much has been written on the death of Libby Zion and the subsequent legal case. The resources I most relied on to retell these stories included *The Girl Who Died Twice* (New York: Delacorte Press, 1995) by Natalie Robins; and *When Illness Goes Public* (Baltimore: The Johns Hopkins University Press, 2006) by Barron H. Lerner, specifically Chapter 10: "You Murdered My Daughter: Libby Zion and the Reform of Medical Education." Both proved very valuable and excellent pieces of reporting and analysis. Additionally, I relied on frequent coverage from *The New York Times;* Craig Horowitz, "The Doctor Is Out," *New York* Magazine, October 27, 2003; David A. Asch and Ruth M. Parker, "Sounding Board: The Libby Zion Case: One Step Forward or Two Steps Backward," *New England Journal of Medicine* 318, no. 12 (March 24, 1998). Most details in this section come from these sources unless otherwise noted.

106   **Sidney would later mote that none of the "pros" had been there:** Sidney Zion, on *Charlie Rose,* July 22, 1993. In recounting the period of his daughter's death, Zion told Rose, "The hospitals then were run by the interns and the residents at night. If you went in on a weekend, which is when it happened, on a Sunday, the pros weren't around."

107   **"an indictment of American graduate Medical Education":** David A. Asch and Ruth M. Parker, "Sounding Board: The Libby Zion Case: One Step Forward or Two Steps Backward," *New England Journal of Medicine* 318, no. 12 (March 24, 1998).

108 **"recommendations were motivated by a desire to improve hospital care":** Ibid.

108 **a number Bell and a colleague came up with while sitting on his porch one day:** Bell relayed this anecdote years later in two different pieces of writing: Bertrand M. Bell, "Reconsideration of the New York State Laws Rationalizing the Supervision and the Working Conditions of Residents," *Einstein Journal of Biology and Medicine* 20, no. 1 (2003); and in a letter to the editor entitled "Resident Duty Hour Reform and Mortality in Hospitalized Patients," *JAMA* 298, no. 24 (December 26, 2007).

109 **An inspection of New York hospitals:** Edward E. Whang et. al., "Implementing Resident Work Hour Limitations," *Annals of Surgery* 237, no. 4 (April 2003).

109 ***Time* magazine ran a piece:** Claudia Wallis, "Re-Examining the 36-Hour Day," *Time,* June 24, 2001.

109 **filed a petition with the U.S. Department of Labor in 2001:** The Health Research Group, "Petition to the Occupational Safety and Health Administration Requesting That Limits Be Placed on Hours Worked by Medical Residents," HRG Publication #1570, April 30, 2001. The petition can be viewed online at http://www.citizen.org/publications/release.cfm?ID=6771.

109 **Representative John Conyers Jr.:** Jason van Steenburgh, "Under Pressure, Medicine Revisits Resident Work Hours," *ACP–ASIM Observer*—The American College of Physicians–American Society of Internal Medicine, March 2002.

109 **the council set limits on hours for residency programs:** Accreditation Council for Graduate Medicine Education (ACGME), "Report of the ACGME Work Group on Resident Duty Hours," June 11, 2002. This report is available online at http://www.acgme.org/DutyHours/wkgroupreport611.pdf.

110　**a *Journal of the American Medical Association* study showed that 83 percent of the interns surveyed:** Christopher P. Landrigan et al., "Interns' Compliance with Accreditation Council for Graduate Medical Education Work-Hour Limits," *JAMA* 296, no. 9 (September 6, 2006).

114　**they routinely drove back to the hospital and only then logged the hours toward the eighty-hour limit:** Accreditation Council for Graduate Medicine Education (ACGME), "Report of the ACGME Work Group on Resident Duty Hours," June 11, 2002. Line 33: "When residents take call from home and are called into the hospital, the time spent in the hospital must be counted toward the weekly duty hour limit."

7: The Other Important Match in Their Lives

139　**Danbury held only 371 beds:** The number of beds available at Danbury Hospital is available online at http://www.danburyhospital.org/body.cfm?id=31.

141　***The New England Journal of Medicine* noted that the number of first births:** Linda J. Heffner, "Advanced Maternal Age—How Old Is Too Old?" *New England Journal of Medicine* 351, no. 19 (November 4, 2004).

144　**A study published in the *Annals of Internal Medicine* four years before:** Virginia U. Collier, "Stress in Medical Residency: Status Quo After a Decade of Reform?" *Annals of Internal Medicine* 136, no. 5 (March 5, 2002).

144　**the average age of a first-time mother in the United States:** "The average age at first birth for U.S. women was 25.2 years in 2005." Joyce A. Martin et al., "Births: Final Data for 2005," *National Vital Statistics Report* 56, no. 6 (December 5, 2007).

145　**national average of less than 28 percent female surgical residents:** AMA Table 4: Women Residents by Specialty 2005. Statistics from *JAMA* 269, no. 9 (September 6, 2006). The table is available online at http://www.ama-assn.org/ama/pub/category/12915.html.

Notes

8: The Intangible Qualities

167 **"embarrassing rubbish" and a "shameless piece of sentimentality":** David Denby, "The Film File: Patch Adams," *New Yorker,* 1999.

10: Finding Time for a Life

204 *Loving the Self-Absorbed: How to Create a More Satisfying Relationship with a Narcissistic Partner,* by Nina W. Brown (Oakland, Calif.: New Harbinger Publications, 2003).

204 *Doctors' Marriages: A Look at the Problems and Their Solutions,* by Michael F. Myers (New York: Springer, 1994).

204 **"Relationship Skills for the Surgical Marriage":** As mentioned in Eddie L. Hoover, "Mentoring Surgeons in Private and Academic Practice," *Archives of Surgery* 140, no. 6 (June 2005).

205 **"How to Survive Your Husband's Residency,"** by Karen Van Buren, "Spouses Corner," *Resident & Staff Physician* S:33(3), March 1987.

205 **medical specialties and divorce:** Bruce L. Rollman, "Medical Specialty and the Incidence of Divorce," *New England Journal of Medicine* 336, no. 11 (March 13, 1997).

206 *Hippocrates' Handmaidens,* by Esther M. Nitzberg (New York: Routledge, 1991).

206 **"Top Ten Tips for Surviving Residency—From a Male Medical Spouse and Father,"** by Brandon Knight. Posted on the MomMD.com Web site as part of his series The Other Side of Medicine.

206 **Dr. Wayne Sotile suggested:** As quoted by Wayne Thompson, "Combat Mentality Helps Medical Marriages Survive," *Wake Forest University News Service.* Posted April 17, 1997. Available online at http://www.wfu .edu/wfunews/1997/041797j.htm.

207 **bringing high returns for its endowment:** Jesse Oxfeld, "Slice of Cheese Pizza at Tresidder Union: $2.75. Econ 1 Textbook: $123.56. Undergraduate Tuition: $29,847. Bloomingdale's Across the Street . . . Priceless," *Stanford Magazine,* July/August 2004.

209 **former U.S. surgeon general C. Everett Koop wrote:** C. Everett Koop, "Marriage and Residency—Incompatible!" Letter to the editor, *The Pharos* 64, no. 1 (winter 2001).

11: One Year Down, the Rest of Their Lives to Go

221 **the Match had continued to grow:** For details on the 2007 Match, see NRMP Press Release, "Record Number of U.S. Medical School Seniors Apply to Residency Programs," March 15, 2007.

230 **in 2003, Bertrand Bell:** Bertrand M. Bell, "Reconsideration of the New York State Laws Rationalizing the Supervision and the Working Conditions of Residents," *Einstein Journal of Biology and Medicine* 20, no. 1 (2003).

231 **House Committee on Energy and Commerce signed a letter:** March 29, 2007. A copy of the letter can be found online at http:// energycommerce.house.gov/Press_110/110-ltr.032907.HHS.Munier.pdf.

231 **the Institute of Medicine had formed a committee:** The Institute of Medicine, "Optimizing Graduate Medical Trainee (Resident) Hours and Work Schedules to Improve Patient Safety." Available online at http:// www.iom.edu/CMS/3809/48553.aspx.

231 **welcoming remarks to the committee:** Remarks by Carolyn M. Clancy, M.D., Director, Agency for Healthcare Research and Quality (AHRQ), "Committee on Optimizing Graduate Medical Trainee (Resident) Hours and Work Schedules," December 3, 2007. Available online at http://www.ahrq .gov/news/sp120307.htm.

Notes

231 **rumors spread among residents in online chat forums and blogs:** Among the blogs and chatrooms where I read discussions of these rumors were Web sites entitled "Forum.Studentdoctor.net," "Kevinmd.com," and "Medschoolhell.com," all accessed on June 16, 2008.

232 **others closer to the committee predicted unlikely:** "Residents Expecting to Work Fewer Hours: Committee May Just Recommend Better Naps." Posted on *The Scalpel* blog on Cleveland.com, Wednesday, May 28, 2008.

232 **An article in the American College of Surgeons' *Surgery News* noted that its own task force:** Jane Anderson, "ACS Urges IOM to Weight Impact of Fewer Duty Hours in the Future," *Surgery News*, June 2008.

232 **Medical school tuition:** Information on tuition and debt came from the Association of American Medical Colleges, "Medical School Tuition and Young Physician Indebtedness: An Update to the 2004 Report," October 2007.

232 **moonlighting:** Sources on moonlighting included the following: Larry Stevens, "Before You Moonlight: The Ins and Outs," *American Medical News,* October 22/29, 2007; Christine Kuehn Kelly, "Moonlighting: Good Experience or a Necessary Evil," *ACP–ASIM Observer*, The American College of Physicians–American Society of Internal Medicine, May 2000; Joshua S. Coren, "Is Moonlighting Right for You?" *Family Practice Management* 14, no. 3 (March 2007), Audiey Kao, "Moonlighting for Charity," *Virtual Mentor* 5, no. 3 (March 2003); "Survey of Moonlighting Practices and Work Requirements of Emergency Medicine Residents," *American Journal of Emergency Medicine* 18, no. 2 (2000): 147–51; "Ethics Poll," *Virtual Mentor* 5, no. 3 (March 2003).